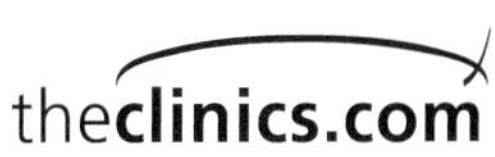

NURSING CLINICS OF NORTH AMERICA

Oncology Nursing: Past, Present, and Future

GUEST EDITORS
Marilyn Frank-Stromborg, MS, EdD, JD, FAAN
Judith Johnson, PhD, RN, FAAN

CONSULTING EDITOR
Suzanne S. Prevost, PhD, RN

June 2008 • Volume 43 • Number 2

SAUNDERS

An Imprint of Elsevier, Inc.
PHILADELPHIA LONDON TORONTO MONTREAL SYDNEY TOKYO

W.B. SAUNDERS COMPANY
A Division of Elsevier Inc.

1600 John F. Kennedy Blvd., Suite 1800, Philadelphia, PA 19103-2899

http://www.theclinics.com

NURSING CLINICS OF NORTH AMERICA
June 2008
Editor: Ali Gavenda

Volume 43, Number 2
ISSN 0029-6465
ISBN-13: 978-1-4160-5777-2
ISBN-10: 1-4160-5777-3

Nursing Clinics of North America (ISSN 0029-6465) is published quarterly by Elsevier Inc., 360 Park Avenue South, New York, NY 10010-1710. Months of issue are March, June, September, and December. Business and Editorial Offices: 1600 John F. Kennedy Blvd., Suite 1800, Philadelphia, PA 19103-2899. Customer Service Office: 6277 Sea Harbor Drive, Orlando, FL 32887-4800. Periodicals postage paid at New York, NY and additional mailing offices. Subscription price per year is, $123.00 (US individuals), $242.00 (US institutions), $198.00 (international individuals), $290.00 (international institutions), $170.00 (Canadian individuals), $290.00 (Canadian institutions), $65.00 (US students), and $100.00 (international students). To receive student/resident rate, orders must be accompanied by name of affiliated institution, date of term, and the signature of program/residency coordinator on institution letterhead. Orders will be billed at individual rate until proof of status is received. Foreign air speed delivery is included in all *Clinics* subscription prices. All prices are subject to change without notice. **POSTMASTER:** Send address changes to *Nursing Clinics*, Elsevier Periodicals Customer Service, 6277 Sea Harbor Drive, Orlando, FL 32887-4800. **Customer Service: 1-800-654-2452 (US). From outside the United States, call 1-407-563-6020. Fax: 1-407-363-9661. E-mail: JournalsCustomerService-usa@elsevier.com**.

Nursing Clinics of North America is covered in *EMBASE/Excerpta Medica, Index Medicus, Social Sciences Citation Index, Current Contents, ASCA, Cumulative Index to Nursing, RNdex Top 100*, and *Allied Health Literature and International Nursing Index (INI).*

Printed in the United States of America.

CONSULTING EDITOR

SUZANNE S. PREVOST, PhD, RN, Nursing Professor and National HealthCare Chair of Excellence, School of Nursing, Middle Tennessee State University, Murfreesboro, Tennessee

GUEST EDITORS

MARILYN FRANK-STROMBORG, MS, EdD, JD, FAAN, Licensed Adult Nurse Practitioner; DeKalb County Drug Court Coordinator; and DeKalb County State's Attorney's Office, Sycamore, Illinois

JUDITH JOHNSON, PhD, RN, FAAN, Nurse Consultant, HealthQuest; and Associate Director, Multinational Association of Supportive Care in Cancer

CONTRIBUTORS

MATTHEW J. BEELEN, MD, Department of Family and Community Medicine, Lancaster General Hospital, Lancaster, Pennsylvania

HARVEY J. COHEN, MD, Geriatrics Division, Duke University School of Medicine; Geriatric Research, Education, and Clinical Center, Veterans Affairs Medical Center; and Center for the Study of Aging and Human Development, Geriatrics Division, Duke University Medical Center, Durham, North Carolina

GEORGIA M. DECKER, MS, APRN-BC, CN, AOCN, Integrative Care, N.P., P.C., Albany, New York

THOMAS J. GATES, MD, Department of Family and Community Medicine, Lancaster General Hospital, Lancaster, Pennsylvania

BARBARA HOLMES GOBEL, RN, MS, AOCN, Oncology Clinical Nurse Specialist, Northwestern Memorial Hospital, Chicago; and Western Springs, Illinois

JOYCE P. GRIFFIN-SOBEL, PhD, RN, AOCN, APRN-BC, CNE, Director, Undergraduate Programs and Associate Professor, Hunter-Bellevue School of Nursing, Hunter College, New York, New York

PAMELA J. HAYLOCK, PhD(c), RN, Doctoral Candidate, The University of Texas Medical Branch, Galveston; and Cancer Care Consultant, Medina, Texas

CURTIS L. HERSHEY, MD, Department of Family and Community Medicine, Lancaster General Hospital, Lancaster, Pennsylvania

SUSAN A. LEIGH, BSN, RN, Cancer Survivorship Consultant and Founding Member, National Coalition for Cancer Survivorship, Tucson, Arizona

DAWN SAWRUN, MSN, APRN-BC, FNP, OCN, Nurse Practitioner and Nursing Educator, The Connecticut Hospice, Branford, Connecticut

LISA SCHULMEISTER, RN, MN, APRN-BC, OCN, FAAN, Self-employed Oncology Nursing Consultant, River Ridge, Louisiana

KAREN J. STANLEY, RN, MSN, AOCN, FAAN, Clinical Nurse Specialist, Pain and Palliative Care Service, Stamford Hospital, Stamford, Connecticut

MARIANNE TREANTAFILOS, MSN, APRN, Co-Director, Nursing and Education, The Connecticut Hospice, Branford, Connecticut

HEIDI K. WHITE, MD, MHS, Geriatrics Division, Duke University School of Medicine; and Geriatric Research, Education, and Clinical Center, Veterans Affairs Medical Center, Durham, North Carolina

CONTENTS

medicine. Complementary and alternative medicine has been referred to as "integrative," "integrated," or "complementary" when therapies are combined with conventional approaches, such as those for cancer.

The Changing Legacy of Cancer: Issues of Long-Term Survivorship **243**
Susan A. Leigh

Although successes in treating cancer have dramatically increased the sheer numbers of survivors, these advancements have outpaced the availability to deliver adequate and responsible follow-up care. Multiple needs of cancer survivors, met and unmet, have been identified, as have several barriers to the delivery of follow-up care. Meanwhile, resources are increasing. Models of care are being developed. Collaboration is replacing competition. Survivors, along with their loved ones and health care providers, continue to work for better access to quality cancer care.

Ethical Issues and Clinical Expertise at the End of Life **259**
Karen J. Stanley, Dawn Sawrun, and Marianne Treantafilos

Oncology care has changed markedly in the past decade. With new therapies, patients are experienced in living with life-threatening illness and believe in the abilities of science and the health care system to find new therapies. Changes in the treatment paradigm have altered oncology nursing practice. The integration of newer targeted therapies with their specific side-effect profiles also has changed end-of-life care. Strategies used to manage patients during the active treatment phase of illness can inform and improve nursing practice when active care has been set aside. Evidence-based practice provides a guide to identify, critically appraise, and use evidence to solve clinical problems.

War on Cancer: Victory or Defeat? **277**
Joyce P. Griffin-Sobel

In 1971, President Nixon launched the "War on Cancer." Oncology professionals proclaim the War has been won. But gaps in cancer care—poor colonoscopy screening rates and technique, prostate cancer surgeries by inexperienced physicians, patients unable to obtain medications, and health care access disparities—make it difficult to support the contention of victory. Research is needed in many areas: the role of environmental exposures in development of cancer, evidence-based cancer prevention strategies, and modifiable risk factors. Policy is needed to address disparities in care. The War on Cancer has not been won: advances have been made, but there is work to be done.

A PHYSICIAN'S PERSPECTIVE

FORTHCOMING ISSUES

September 2008

Vulnerable Populations
Marcia K. Stanhope, DSN, RN, FAAN, Lisa M. Turner, MSN, APRN, BC, and Peggy Riley, RN, MSN, *Guest Editors*

December 2008

Technology Use in Nursing Education
Betsy Weiner, PhD, RN, BC, FAAN, *Guest Editor*

March 2009

Evidence-Based Practice
Alyce A. Schultz, RN, PhD, FAAN, *Guest Editor*

RECENT ISSUES

March 2008

Biology, Psychology, and Behavior in Cardiovascular and Pulmonary Disease
Susan K. Frazier, PhD, RN, Terry A. Lennie, PhD, RN, and Debra K. Moser, DNSc, RN, FAAN, *Guest Editors*

December 2007

Sexuality and Chronic Illness: Assessment and Interventions
Margaret C. Wilmoth, PhD, MSS, RN, *Guest Editor*

September 2007

Dermatologic Nursing
Heather Jones, RN, BSN, *Guest Editor*

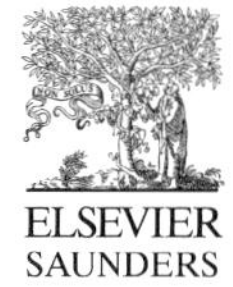

NURSING CLINICS OF NORTH AMERICA

Nurs Clin N Am 43 (2008) ix–xii

Preface

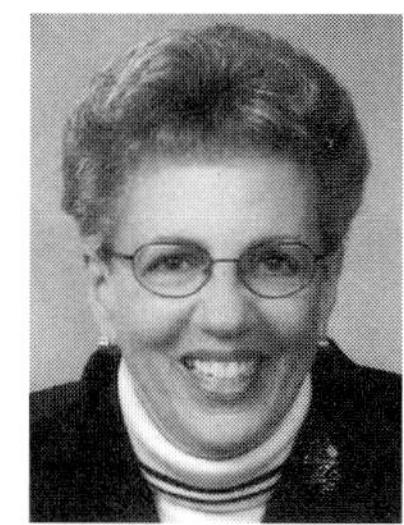

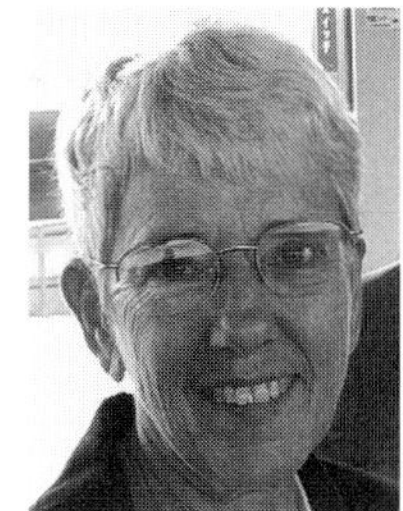

Marilyn Frank-Stromborg, MS, EdD, JD, FAAN

Judith Johnson, PhD, RN, FAAN

Guest Editors

The progress made in cancer treatment and care over the past centuries has been minor when compared to the rapid changes in cancer treatment of the past three decades. Discovery of new drugs, novel treatment delivery systems, advancements in technologies, and more quality research have radically changed the "face of cancer." Today, oncology nursing is a highly regarded nursing specialty and the Oncology Nursing Society has over 36,000 members. Perhaps, the most important change of all is that cancer has moved from being a disease from which you die to one with which you learn to live. Improvements in screening practices and rates, early detection, and cancer treatment and care are allowing more and more people to live "beyond" cancer each year. There are more then 11 million cancer survivors in the United States and another 1.5 million will be diagnosed in 2008 [1].

Today we talk about cancer as a "chronic illness" and cancer patients as "cancer survivors." Nurses are being called upon to meet and care for these individuals in every health care setting. Changes in treatment and management of cancer have created both new challenges and opportunities for nurses. The topics in this issue of *Clinics* highlight many of these changes, along with the rationale for why oncology nurses should lead the way in providing quality cancer care.

This issue of *Nursing Clinics of North America* features articles by nurse educators, practitioners, and researchers who are experts in the field of oncology nursing. The authors are also national leaders in the Oncology Nursing Society, the largest cancer nursing organization in the world. For

doi:10.1016/j.cnur.2008.03.002

example, Georgia Decker is the President, and Pam Haylock (1997–1998) and Karen Stanley (2004–2006) are past-presidents. Lisa Schulmeister (2005–2008) and Barbara Holmes Gobel (2007–2010) are presently on the Oncology Nursing Society's Board of Directors. The authors of this edition have contributed articles in the areas of cancer nursing in which they are recognized experts.

We have selected topics for this issue to be representative of the field of oncology nursing, with particular attention given to emerging and sometimes controversial issues. For example, questions posed include: Is the war on cancer being won? What role do alternative cancer therapies have in the treatment of cancer? What are the ethical issues that are typically encountered when caring for someone in the end of life? And, what issues have evolved with long-term cancer survivorship? In addition, we selected topics about which we know nurses have significant clinical involvement and vested interest.

Pam Haylock presents a comprehensive history of cancer nursing in general and specifically in the United States. Most importantly, she discusses the issues that will emerge with contemporary oncology nursing, as well as the future of the profession. Ms. Haylock points out that the contemporary domain of cancer nursing has an undeniable, long, and rich history. "A desire to make a difference for people facing the challenges of cancer has been and remains the essence of cancer nursing" (Haylock, p. 198).

Symptom management has always been a focus of oncology nursing. Lisa Schulmeister and Barbara Holmes Gobel present the concept of symptom clusters versus a single symptom. Symptom clusters are defined as two or more symptoms that are related to each other and occur together. These authors argue that symptom burden may be an effective approach to investigating the late and long-term effects of cancer treatment. It is postulated that using the concept of symptom burden may be a more effective method of invcstigation than thc usc of singlc-symptom or quality of lifc. Against the discussion of symptom clusters and symptom burden, they present arguments that evidence-based guidelines need to be disseminated and their clinical use encouraged.

It wasn't until the late 1990s that alternative medicines achieved acceptance in the medical community. In 1998, the National Center for Complementary and Alternative Medicine was founded, which is one of 27 institutes that make up the National Institutes of Health. In the same year, the National Cancer Institute (NCI) established the Office of Cancer Complementary and Alternative Medicine within the office of the Director. Georgia Decker details the commonly used Complementary and Alternative Medicines (CAMs), such as acupuncture, Reiki, herbal products, shark and bovine cartilage, antioxidants, and the clinical trials that are testing these products. She also details the CAMs that are used in symptom management and the role of the nurse in the administration of CAMs.

Another newly emerging area is cancer survivorship. Susan Leigh is credited as the nurse who is responsible for bringing this area to national attention. It has been two decades since Leigh and other advocates created a new social movement by teaming the concept of survivorship with cancer. How the picture of survivorship has changed is illustrated by the fact that in 1971, there were 3 million cancer survivors and now there are almost 25 million worldwide. In 1995, the Office of Cancer Survivorship was established at the NCI. Ms. Leigh points out that presently there is an identified need for survivorship guidelines and care plans, along with issues of who will take care of them and how.

Also emerging in the past decade is care of the cancer patient at the end of life and the ethical issues and required clinical expertise during this time. Stanley, Sawrun, and Treantafilos offer a multitude of areas that raise ethical concerns at the end of life. These include truth telling, withholding or withdrawing treatment, and requests for assistance in dying. The authors don't stop at presenting the ethical issues the nurse will encounter during this time, but also identify the symptoms that occur at the end of life. They present an in-depth discussion of clinical nursing approaches to help alleviate or ameliorate these symptoms. Throughout their presentation, the need to increase the autonomy of the patients is stressed. Ms. Stanley and her colleagues stress that protocols must be in place to assure autonomy, informed consent, technical expertise, and ongoing interdisciplinary and family or caregiver communication.

Since President Nixon launched the "War on Cancer" in 1971, literally billions of dollars have been spent on the disease cancer. The question posed by Griffin-Sobel is whether or not the progress in cancer care and treatment merits saying that the war has been won. While there have been declines in cancer mortality rates and dramatic advances made in the treatment of many cancers, does this equal victory over the disease?

In the article on cancer screening in men, Gates, Beelen, and Hershey argue that the experience of cancer screening is different for men and women. The general considerations in screening are discussed and include the benefits and harms of screening and bias in the evaluation of screening tests. Lastly, the epidemiology of cancer in men, along with the current screening controversies associated with each type of cancer, are discussed.

Finally, in their article on the older cancer patient, White and Cohen point out that more than half of cancers occur in adults over the age of 65 years. They advocate the use of a comprehensive geriatric assessment (CGA) by health care professionals (nurses, social workers, and midlevel practitioners) to evaluate older patients who have cancer to improve the care of this population. The CGA can be used to tailor treatment for individual patients and establish goals of care.

We would like to thank the nurses and their contributing coauthors, who generously gave their time and talents to the creation of this issue. We would also like to thank Ali Gavenda, Editor of *Nursing Clinics of North America*, for recognizing the need to have an edition devoted exclusively to oncology nursing and the importance of this topic to nurses. This issue does not attempt to be comprehensive in nature or scope; rather, it attempts to focus on topics that are currently impacting the clinical practice of nurses. It is expected that nurses will use this information to improve their practice and develop or expand their programs of research.

Marilyn Frank-Stromborg, MS, EdD, JD, FAAN
Licensed Adult Nurse Practitioner
DeKalb County Drug Court Coordinator
133 West State Street
Sycamore, IL 60178, USA

DeKalb County State's Attorney's Office
200 North Main Street
Sycamore, IL 60178, USA

E-mail addresses: mstromborg@dekalbcounty.org; cancer@niu.edu

Judith Johnson, PhD, RN, FAAN
Nurse Consultant
HealthQuest
Associate Director
Multinational Association of Supportive Care in Cancer

E-mail address: judibj@comcast.net

Reference

[1] Mayer D. Does everyone with cancer need an oncology nurse? Clin J of Oncol Nurs 2008; 12(1):11.

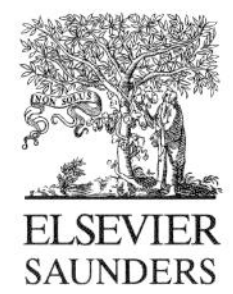

ELSEVIER
SAUNDERS

Nurs Clin N Am 43 (2008) 179–203

NURSING
CLINICS
OF NORTH AMERICA

Cancer Nursing: Past, Present, and Future

Pamela J. Haylock, PhD(c), RN[a,b]

[a]*The University of Texas Medical Branch, 301 University Boulevard, Galveston, TX 77555, USA*
[b]*Cancer Care Consultant, 18954 State Highway 16 North, Medina, TX 78055, USA*

From the beginning of recorded history, cancer has been a disease laden with myths, misconceptions, and valid fears. Until well into the twentieth century, most cancer diagnoses were universally fatal. When a group of physicians met in 1913 to establish the American Society for the Control of Cancer, forerunner of the American Cancer Society, they did so in a New York City brownstone with shades pulled: physicians who had any kind of repute could ill afford to risk their careers by being associated with such a nefarious activity [1]. Nevertheless, America's War on Cancer had been declared [2]. Despite the dismal circumstances, nurses—trained and lay—provided care for people who had cancer, and a few emerged in the late nineteenth and early twentieth centuries to provide a foundation for a recognized and strong nursing specialty. The contributions of many of these nurses are well documented in available resources, including cancer nursing texts [3], reference books [4–6], and materials from the Oncology Nursing Society (ONS) [1,7,8]. What is not so widely available is primary source material documenting clinical nursing practice of nurses throughout history who have quietly and almost inconspicuously provided essential care for people who have had cancer—nurses who Lusk [9,10] refers to as the collectively "overlooked soldiers in the cancer wars." But these historically overlooked nurses, together with often-cited leaders, integrated complex personal, societal, political, scientific, and technologic realities of their times into a legacy of scholarship, professionalism, social justice, and ingenuity that continues today to characterize cancer nursing. This article provides an overview of the historical context, a glimpse of clinical cancer nursing through the ages, a look at contemporary cancer nursing at the beginning of the twenty-first century, and musings about the future of this continuously evolving professional nursing specialty.

E-mail address: pjhaylock@indian-creek.net

doi:10.1016/j.cnur.2008.02.003 *nursing.theclinics.com*

The historical context of cancer nursing

Cancer nursing emerged as a specialty requiring education beyond basic nursing in the United States in the early 1940s [9–11] and gained momentum after President Nixon signed the National Cancer Act in 1971 [12]. But humans knew and feared cancer before Hippocrates. The Edwin Smith Papyrus from Egypt, dating to the seventeenth century BC, provides the oldest written description of a person who had a malignant tumor, concluding, "there is no treatment" [13]. Hippocrates, Celsus, and Galen set a pattern for cancer care that remained for centuries, relying on methods to "soothe the tumor" [13] rather than developing methods to control, cure, or remove it [14]. During the Dark Ages (AD 476–1200), care was provided by female herbalists and "wise women," relying on therapies derived from botanicals, home remedies, purges, and bloodletting [15]. Nursing care was the predominant service, providing the comforts of "bed, board, bath, and prayer" [15]. By the eighteenth century, descriptions of surgical procedures for cancer emerged. The first abdominal operations were gynecologic procedures: the first ovariotomy was performed in 1809 on patient Jane Todd Crawford by Dr. Ephraim McDowell, known as the father of abdominal surgery [16]. Mrs. Crawford submitted to the surgery, without anesthesia, after riding 60 miles on horseback to reach Dr. McDowell's home in Danville, Kentucky, "resting the tumor on the horn of her saddle" [2,16]. Mrs. Crawford survived the operation, escaped the onset of infection, returned home in 25 days, and lived another 33 years [16]. (A 22-bed hospital in Greensburg, Kentucky, is named for the pioneer heroine of abdominal surgery—the Jane Todd Crawford Memorial Hospital.) Another century passed before surgical anesthesia, aseptic practices, and antibiotic therapy allowed the development and more routine use of radical operations, such as the classic radical mastectomy [14] and abdominal perineal resection [17,18].

The emergence of cancer nursing

Informal and formal cancer nursing occurs within the context of the state of medical science and technology, social norms, interactions between the medical and nursing disciplines, and the evolutionary stage of professional nursing. The first contagious disease hospital for cancer opened in Rheims, France, in 1740, reflecting professional and public debate over the notion of cancer as an infectious disease [19]. The belief in the vegetable origin of cancer was common [20]. In the early twentieth century, "nurses had flatly refused to take charge of cancer cases, on account of the supposed danger to themselves" [21] and suspicions that cancer was a contagious disease were entrenched well into the 1930s [22].

The first hospitals in the United States were established in the mid-eighteenth century to provide nursing care for sick and poor working class citizens [23]. Care for the sick occurred primarily in homes, was provided largely by female family members, and was guided by family traditions and advice published in medical and nursing manuals of the day [24,25]. Families who could afford to do so hired doctors and nurses to provide care in patients' homes with assistance provided by female family members, servants, and neighbors [24]. Those who could not afford to hire caregivers were left to depend on haphazard charitable services or faced the prospect of almshouses where little or no skilled care was offered [23,25].

The desperate situation of the "cancerous poor" in the late nineteenth century provided the catalyst for Rose Hawthorne Lathrop (1851–1926) to become an early advocate of skilled and compassionate care for poor people afflicted with cancer [7,26–28]. Mrs. Lathrop learned of a young seamstress who had become ill with cancer. After spending her savings searching for a cure, the young woman died in despair and her body was dumped in a pauper's grave, not an unusual end for the "cancerous poor" [7,26]. Hospital beds were not available to these people, and most were "left to rot and die in damp cellars or wherever they found a space to crawl into" [7]. Mrs. Lathrop founded the Servants of Relief for Incurable Cancer of the Congregation of St. Rose of Lima, part of the Dominican Third Order, eventually taking the name, Mother Mary Alphonsa. She established her own cancer hospital, St. Rose's Free Home, in 1899 [27,28]. Today, six homes in the United States (in Manhattan and Hawthorne in New York; Philadelphia; Atlanta; St. Paul; and Parma, Ohio) carry on the work of Mother Alphonsa, providing cancer care for the poor without charge [26].

An article submitted by Miss J.C. Sleet, "a young colored woman and a trained nurse," to the *American Journal of Nursing* (*AJN*) in its first year of publication [29], alludes to her sensitivity to cultural influences on her patients' needs. After training at the Providence Hospital "for colored patients" in Chicago, Miss Sleet went to New York to work among "the neglected ones of her own race" [29]. She bathed patients, applied poultices, dressed wounds, and instructed family caregivers, as would any district nurse of her day. But, she felt it necessary to comment on the impact of her race on her ability to meet her patients' needs:

> I cannot but feel that this house-to-house visiting, these face-to-face practical talks, which I am having with the people, must bring about good results. They have welcomed me to their homes, saying, "We don't know you, but we belong to the same race" [30].

From homes to hospitals

Between 1870 and 1920, hospitals became the center of medical education and practice in America, nursing emerged as a trained profession, the nature of hospitals' business and services drastically changed, and the primary settings for care of the sick moved from homes to hospitals. The acceptance of Lister's antisepsis methods and improved infection control meant that surgeons were able to perform more daring surgical procedures for an increasing variety of conditions. The greater volume of surgical work was the basis for expansion of hospital care and its profits. Whereas in earlier times, sick people entered and stayed in hospitals for the entire duration of an illness, the sick now entered hospitals during acute stages of illness, underwent diagnostic and surgical procedures, and left the hospital when improving health status was apparent [25]. Hospital revenues previously generated by charging for home-based services performed by student nurses diminished as the twentieth century progressed. Hospital-based home care nearly disappeared in the face of more lucrative inpatient services. Student nurses, a source of free labor for hospitals that had schools of nursing, provided care for the growing population of paying inpatients [24]. Trained, graduate nurses were self-employed primarily as private duty nurses. Many hospitals continued to refuse patients who had cancer, paying or not, through the first decade of twentieth-century America, primarily because of hospitals' focus on curable patients rather than chronic invalids [10,25].

America's first cancer hospitals emerged between 1884 and 1950. One outcome of designated cancer hospitals was student nurses' exposure to concentrated populations of patients who had cancer. In an attempt to uncover the clinical practice of "ordinary nurses" [9] and student nurses in the care of people who had cancer from 1880 to 1950, Lusk found that nurses' notes in patients' medical charts routinely were destroyed as charts were prepared for storage [9]. Lusk [10] also noted that during this time, physicians authored the majority of journal articles and books published about cancer nursing.

Dr. Goethe Link, Assistant Professor of Gynecology at the Indiana University School of Medicine, addressed the Indiana State Nurses' Association in 1911 and his remarks were published in the *AJN* [31]. He described the heroic work of the nurse who assisted his surgeon father as he performed a laparotomy in rustic southern Indiana in the late 1800s. The patient developed pneumonia, and "alternating shifts for sleep, nurse and surgeon held the patient like a babe for days and nights to keep her from coughing out the stitches" [31]. Maintenance of surgical asepsis was essential, and the nurse was charged with many tasks including cleansing of sponges and instruments, along with "constant attention of a faithful and trained nurse" [31] to early forms of drainage. He spoke of the "insufficiently remembered importance" [31] of trained nurses in this period of medical development:

> Indiana is overrun with so-called nurses, many of whom have never been in a training school at all or only for an incomplete course. The people do not know the difference between the untrained nurse and the competent nurse.... Frequently I am called to operate in the home at a distance from a hospital. Usually, I am told not to bring a nurse, that one has already been engaged. Upon arriving I find, to my dismay, one who has been in a hospital three months and has been dismissed, or one who is

> a graduate of a correspondence school. Her knowledge usually consists of wearing the cap and gown and looking like a trained nurse. She has entrenched herself before I arrive and I must treat her with deference. Her desire to show her skill, together with unfamiliarity with asepsis, makes her dangerous. A sick patient requiring laparotomy and an ignorant nurse make about all one man can handle [31].

Although not specific to cancer nurses, debate over 8-hour versus 12-hour days in schools of nursing and subsequently in hospital work was introduced to *AJN* readers in 1919 [32]. Arguments considered not only the mental and physical taxing on students induced by 12-hour shifts but also the notion of potential conflict between traditions of nursing history and obligations of a profession.

Nurse-authored articles began to appear with more frequency in the 1930s. Letters and other columns routinely included in the *AJN* provide glimpses into the everyday contributions of nurses caring for patients who had cancer. People who had cancer increasingly received nursing care in hospitals. Cancer nursing of the time was perceived as consisting "of nothing but hard, depressing work with failure at the end" [33], as the majority of patients had advanced disease. Finding early-stage cancers was uncommon and the death rate exceeded 90%. Women were socialized to believe it was indecent to bring gynecologic conditions to light, that people would link such conditions with carelessness, wickedness, and venereal disease [34]. Other myths linked cancer with punishments from God: women believed they had done something wrong to get "*that* kind of cancer—cancer of the womb" [1]. The stigma and resultant humiliation attached to various forms of cancer contributed to deadly delays in diagnosis and, for nurses, the undesirable perception of working with cancer-afflicted persons.

Surgery was the only effective treatment for cancer until the 1940s and then only if the disease was discovered in early and localized stages. People feared surgery with good reason: anesthesia was unpleasant and dangerous, hemorrhage was common, and blood transfusions before blood biology was well understood were traumatic and risky. Death from sepsis was always a distinct possibility in the preantibiotic period [3]. Cancer nursing consisted mostly of traditional bedside care and comfort measures directed by the advanced stage of disease and treatment-related complications. Nurses were forced to use ingenuity and creative skills to address difficult problems, including management of profuse fistulae drainage, odor control, radiation burns, and, of course, pain management [3,35].

Anne Ferris, Director of Nursing at Memorial Hospital, described developments in the nursing care of patients who had cancer in 1930, noting that the "attitude toward cancer nursing is changing" [35]. She described the extensive use of radium and radiographs and the subsequent "new type of inflammation," that caused tissue breakdown, "accumulation of necrotic and sloughing tissue and secondary infection that must be cared for" [35]. She explained hourly irrigation techniques that were applied to sloughing areas of patients who had head and neck cancers. Nurses providing care for patients who had undergone gastrostomy operations were advised in measures to "build up the patient's physical condition to the point where he can be operated upon and after the operation, of feeding him and teaching him, if possible, to feed and care for himself" [35]. Ferris also provided intricate detail—along with photographs—of techniques for tracheotomy care similar to those used by nurses today.

The potential usefulness of radiation—radiographs and radium—was discovered in the late 1800s. Radiation was accepted as a therapeutic option for many forms of superficial cancers by the 1920s, although knowledge of radiobiology was limited [36]. By 1930, it was a nurse's duty to make up all applicators used in radium therapy, and nurses were advised to become familiar with the physics of radioactive materials [37]. Suggested nursing interventions consisted of provision of the essential elements, "rest, diet, fresh air, and proper care of the local lesion" [37]. Foul odor from lesions was addressed by adding a "few drops of bergamot mixed with the ointment applied or sprinkled on the dressing," while "small amounts of iced ginger ale or sodium bicarbonate," it was suggested, could relieve nausea and vomiting [37]. Nurses were asked to become sources of information about prevention, recognition, and care of cancer cases, and public health nurses, in particular, were seen to have an "unusual opportunity for detecting early cases" and able to exert an "intelligent influence on these cases…to induce them to seek immediate and competent treatment" [37]. Nurses were advised of the dangers to themselves associated with the handling of radium and radon and given the precaution that these materials should "never be picked up with the fingers" [37]. A photograph of the fingers of a nurse who had been making radium applicators is included in a 1930 *AJN* article. The caption reads,

> Condition of fingers of nurse who had been making applicators over a period of eighteen months. Note pitted appearance of skin on finger tips, thickened cuticle near nails, and slight ulceration on the second finger. This picture was taken in 1914. Tactile sense at present time [1930] has not returned to normal and nails are still brittle [37].

General handling rules included adoption of a monthly rotation of service for nurses charged with handling applicators. Long-handled forceps were used to move radioactive sources from patients to storage in lead containers placed at a distance from handlers and patients. Blood assessments for leucopenia or mild anemia were to be performed on all workers before starting their duties and thereafter on a monthly basis [37].

Early chemotherapy was limited to caustic agents, including arsenic pastes and Coley's toxins, applied locally, acting by chemically burning away or reducing superficial cancers [38,39]. Between 1865 and 1931, arsenic was used to treat leukemia. During and after World War II, the potential of systemic antitumor drugs was recognized and drugs with greater activity were introduced, including nitrogen mustard, first noted to induce tumor regression in 1942 [39]. Between 1940 and 1950 many drug development programs were devised, and in 1955, the National Cancer Institute (NCI) created the Cancer Chemotherapy National Service Center and development of the clinical trials network [39].

1930 through 1950

By the 1930s, scientific advances were changing health patterns and needs for nursing changed too. As communicable diseases were increasingly controlled, old needs for nursing gave way to new, including caring for persons who had cardiovascular disease and persons who had cancer [40]. By 1930, patients were beginning to understand that they need not be ashamed of having cancer and they sought treatment at earlier stages. Survival time was increased and suffering reduced, and the outlook for people who had cancer was not totally hopeless. It already was clear that "there is a definite field for nurses in the care of these patients, and much of their happiness and comfort depends upon the skill and understanding with which that care is given" [35]. The emotional and psychologic influences on recovery were apparent in the nursing literature. A student nurses' page in a 1938 issue of the *AJN* told readers,

> Fear tires the patient and makes her less resistant to the complications possible after any operation.... The patient will face the operation more calmly if she feels that the nurse is personally interested in her welfare, is capable of giving her the care she needs....The generally run down condition of many patients by the time they enter a hospital makes them poorly equipped to face crises. The doctor cures the physical ills of the patient (with the nurse's aid) but it is up to the nurse to help that patient to become a person once more able to face and cope with life [34].

Nursing educators recognized that the educational philosophy referred to as integration—integrating new information into an otherwise undisturbed curriculum—provided insufficient instruction with regard to cancer nursing. Nursing leader and educator Dr. Katherine Nelson described inadequacies of nursing education curricula with regard to cancer nursing:

> It now seemed quite right and proper to "integrate" a little cancer instruction into all the well established and familiar courses....Unfortunately in many instances this little became very little indeed and some of the major therapies for cancer were dealt with briefly or left out entirely. A little chemotherapy was put into pharmacology but instruction in radiation as a therapy was practically non-existent. Students knew what patients received radiation therapy but had little or no knowledge of why or what to do about it. If the patient's physician wanted something done, he left an order to that effect and that was the end of it [40].

Graduate nurses were well prepared to work in hospitals, but they had limited knowledge of disease control in society or what happened to the patient, family, and the community when a person was afflicted with cancer. In 1942, the Joint Committee of the National Organization for Public Health Nursing and the United States Public Health Service published *The Public Health Nurse Curriculum Guide* [41]. The target learner was a graduate nurse who intended to be a practitioner of nursing not an administrator. Of 16 identified functional areas, one was designated as cancer—something Nelson referred to as "an important historical milestone" [40]—the first time in nursing education history that a part of the curriculum was devoted solely to cancer.

As a Philadelphia visiting nurse in the 1940s, Virginia Barckley (1911–1993) witnessed the suffering of patients and families who faced cancer. By then, survival rates had increased to 25% but radiation and chemotherapy were not considered truly effective therapies until the 1950s. Miss Barckley reflected that at the time, the word "cancer" was largely avoided, and nurses were prohibited from talking with patients and families about diagnosis, prognosis, or details of the illness [5,10], a practice that nurse Johnson [42] referred to as "verging on deceit." The question of disclosure of the cancer diagnosis appears in the nursing literature again and again through the present day [43,44]. Earlier journal articles offered suggestions for how nurses could benignly deceive patients who worried about their diagnosis by "working into her conversation the fact that radiation is used for a wide variety of conditions without even mentioning that cancer is one of them" or, in the event that a patient asked point blank whether or not he had cancer, advising the nurse "to turn the question right back to him by saying, 'What did your doctor tell you was your difficulty?'" [43,44]. Miss Barckley recalled her early cancer nursing days, "You couldn't be a visiting nurse without seeing a great deal of cancer, and you couldn't see a great deal of cancer, especially in the 1940's, without being deeply touched and deeply impressed" [1]. She was an early proponent of cancer nursing as a specific practice domain, defying the commonly held assumptions that cancer nursing was a "grim concatenation of hard work, boredom, and frustration, without even the hope of recovery at the end" [45]. Instead, she reminded us,

> If we fail to perceive the excitement and challenge in cancer nursing, we miss the opportunity, given to so few, to learn the difference our own care can make in enhancing the comfort and the survival of such patients [45].

Miss Barckley was fully cognizant of the discouraging and trying nature of early cancer nursing but suggested, "When revulsion is replaced by compassion, when we think 'What can I do to help?' instead of 'Poor me!' we are functioning on a high level" [46].

Clinical nursing care in the 1940s still consisted primarily of symptom management. Side effects of radiation-induced nausea and vomiting were treated with a mixture of lemon juice, sour wine, and ginger ale [47]. In late stages of cancer, cobra venom, alcohol injections, operations on nerves, and use of radiation were used to keep patients free from excruciating pain [48]. Narcotics generally were reserved for patients who had "access to full care," whereas coal-tar derivatives, aspirin, and codeine were believed useful for more moderate pain. Urea applications were used to decrease the odor of open and draining breast lesions [49].

The science of the 1940s set the stage for advances and "firsts" in cancer nursing. Dr. Nelson referred to the 1940s as the "heyday" for cancer and cancer nursing [40]. The deadly cytotoxic consequences of nitrogen mustard, used in World War I as an agent of gas warfare, were harnessed and used as an effective antineoplastic agent beginning in 1942 [39,50]. A second antineoplastic agent, aminopterin, was used to achieve the first remission, followed by an increasing array of drugs with various mechanisms of action [39]. Advances in prevention and early detection included promotion of breast self-examination and development and implementation of the Papanicolaou smear technique used to identify early cancerous changes in cells of the uterine cervix [3].

The Nursing Section of the Cancer Control Branch of the NCI was created in 1948. Rosalie Peterson was named Senior Nurse Officer and Chief Public Health Nursing Consultant of the Cancer Control Division. Under Peterson's guidance, courses directed toward nursing school faculty were developed and offered to enhance nurses' knowledge of cancer, home care, and rehabilitation [3].

In 1947, Miss Anne Ferris, Director of Nursing at the Memorial Hospital for Cancer and Allied Diseases (now Memorial Sloan-Kettering Cancer Center), collaborated with Dr. Nelson at Teachers College, Columbia University, to offer the first university course in cancer nursing specialization [3,40]. Practicum training was held at Memorial Hospital and practice with patients who had advanced-stage cancers took place at Montefiore Hospital in the Bronx. Field visits and tours were part of the curriculum, including tours of the NCI in Washington, DC, the cancer research center in Bethesda, Maryland, and animal research and other cancer research laboratories. Eventually, the course provided 16 academic credit hours toward a Master of Arts degree.

Miss Renilda Hilkemeyer (1915–2007), known internationally as a pioneer of cancer nursing administration and education, entered cancer nursing in 1950 as a consultant in nursing education in the Bureau of Cancer Control in Missouri. Recognizing the many settings in which people who have cancer require nursing care, Miss Hilkemeyer initiated an educational program in 1950 to teach hospital and nursing school personnel and public health nurses about the care of patients who had cancer [51]. The novel course curriculum, conducted at the Ellis Fischel State Cancer Hospital in Columbia, Missouri, emphasized a multidisciplinary approach to the "social, emotional, and rehabilitation aspects of chronic disease with particular reference to the cancer patient" [51]. In 1955, Miss Hilkemeyer became Director of the Department of Nursing and Professor in Oncology Nursing at the University of Texas System Cancer Center M. D. Anderson Hospital and Tumor Institute in Houston, where she stayed until her retirement in 1977 [6]. At Anderson, Miss Hilkemeyer changed the role of nurses from one in which the nurses were "running around after the doctor...running around with the clipboard or running around taking his orders, sitting at the desk doing all of this stuff..." [8] to expecting nurses to provide direct patient care. She undertook an organizational study that revealed that nurses spent less than 20% of their time with patients and orderlies spent more than 20% of their time off the units [8]. She devised innovations for hospital organization, such as use of ward clerks to transcribe physicians' orders and requiring physicians actually to write their own orders. She reports telling doctors, "Your fun days are over: you are going to start writing your own orders...and start taking care of yourself!" [8], and instituted transportation orderlies, all changes that allowed nurses more time to be with patients. Her skill and contribution were to create an organizational environment in which educated and competent nurses' roles centered on patient care at Anderson, an exemplar for state-of-the-art cancer nursing throughout the world [6].

1950 through 1980

Mid–twentieth century cancer treatment in America consisted of "extensive surgery or massive radiation or intensive hormonal therapy, or a combination of these" [52,53]. Toxicities associated with cancer treatment usually made patients quite ill and in need of highly skilled nursing care. In some settings, nurses operated radiation therapy equipment and provided day-to-day observations, patient self-care instructions, skin care to prevent irritation and infection, nutritional counseling, and other measures to promote "good physical condition and morale" [43,52,54]. The emotional and psychosocial impact of cancer was recognized, culminating in the realizations that nursing performance needed to be improved and that additional preparation was needed to prepare nurses to offer comprehensive care to patients who had cancer [52]. In addition to direct care for persons already sick from cancer, early case finding was perceived as a professional responsibility of all nurses [52].

The American Cancer Society, an organizational champion of cancer nursing throughout its history, formed its Nursing Advisory Committee in 1948 and published the first reference book for nurses, *A Cancer Source Book for Nurses*, in 1950 [55]. The 120-page book contained information about cancer for nurses, providing what was considered good, basic knowledge of the subject. It was available free of charge from state divisions of the American Cancer Society or from its national office. Also in 1950, *Cancer Nursing: A Manual for Public Health Nurses,* was published as a joint project of the NCI, United States Public Health Service, and the New York

State Department of Health [56]. It was available free of charge in New York and sold for $1 in other states. It included an overview of cancer nursing; definitions of terms; descriptions of community programs for detection, diagnosis, and treatment of cancers; and a section on home care procedures, including gastrostomy feeding, colostomy irrigation, tracheotomy care, and arm exercises.

Before 1950, authors of journal articles about nursing of patients who had cancer tended to suggest that the nurse taking care of terminally ill patients should be a "cheerful attendant" [49]. Contrary to the dismal perception of cancer nursing that Barckley described, nurse authors Handorf and Pedersen [57], wrote "Nursing Care in Terminal Cancer" in 1950, suggesting that care of patients who have cancer in terminal stages is "rich in opportunities for comfort to the patient and his family as well as satisfaction to the nurse" [57]. Handorf and Pederson [57] maintained, "expert nursing and application of techniques for terminal care were familiar to nurses in the care of other chronic and progressive diseases" but that special problems "produced by cancer could aggravate ordinary nursing problems." Nurses' special attention, they suggest, should be given to the "maintenance of strength and nutrition, prevention and treatment of bedsores, relief of pain and discomfort, maintenance of aesthetic factors, and provision of occupation and recreation" [57].

Nurse historian Lynaugh [58] refers to the period between 1950 and 1980 as "a time of erratic but fundamental change in every arena of nursing." Certainly this was true in cancer nursing. Internal and external influences on nursing practice were apparent, including the transition from pupil nurse–provided care in hospitals to hospital-employed nurses and changes in nursing education. The Nurse Training Act of 1964 (NTA), a component of President Johnson's Great Society initiatives, indicated that the number and preparation of nurses were central to America's health agenda [58]. Traineeship money encouraged the development of master's degree training programs; applicants got direct aid for tuition and stipends, encouraging nurses to enroll. The NTA was a catalyst for the founding of many specialty nursing organizations in the 1970s, including the Association of Pediatric Oncology Nurses (APON) in 1974 (now the Association of Pediatric/Hematologic Oncology Nurses) and the ONS in 1975.

Contemporary oncology nursing

It has been speculated that oncology nursing and medical oncology owe their development to the expansion of clinical trials in the 1960s [59]. Nurses initially were involved in clinical trial teams as data collectors and were responsible to research physicians. Patient care, observations, and counseling theoretically were functions of house staff physicians under the supervision of clinical investigators. Gradually, the oncology nurse role changed as enrolled trial participants sought continuity in relationships with clinical trial teams and clinical investigators found that research nurses provided better information about patient status. Henke [60] referred to this as a symbiotic relationship between trial doctors and nurses "whose only real special training was acquired on-the-job together." The nursing role expanded beyond task-oriented functions to include serving as liaison between clinical investigators and other disciplines that were becoming common to cancer care teams. Over time, the team model was recognized as a better way to provide cancer care not only in research settings but also in nonresearch and community-based settings [60]. It was acknowledged that patients who have cancer require expert specialty nursing care beyond acute, hospital-based care, including home and hospice settings. Subspecialized nursing roles were identified in radiation oncology, enterostomal therapy, cancer detection, patient education, nursing education, and nursing research [60].

Nursing research and clinical excellence

The expanding interest in cancer nursing is reflected by the emergence of professional journals targeting nursing in the rapidly growing specialty. *Cancer Nursing*: *An International Journal for Cancer Care*, an independent professional journal dedicated solely to the specialty, was first published in 1978, as a "vehicle to document accomplishments in the specialized field of cancer nursing" [61]. In 1983, *Cancer Nursing* forged its formal affiliation with the newly established International Society of Nurses in Cancer Care and continues its tradition of facilitating international presentation of cancer nursing research and clinical care articles [61]. From its inception, the APON published the *APON Newsletter,* expanding to journal format as the *Journal of the Association of Pediatric Oncology Nurses* in 1984 [62]. In 2006, the organization changed its name to the Association of Pediatric Hematology Oncology Nurses, and the journal became the *Journal of the Association of Pediatric Hematology/Oncology Nurses* to better reflect the realities of pediatric cancer care (C. Schmidt, personal communication, December 7, 2007). In 1977, the ONS newsletter transitioned to become the society's official publication, the *Oncology Nursing Forum,* featuring organizational news and clinical and research articles. A second ONS publication, the *Clinical Journal of Oncology Nursing,* began publication in 1997 in response to members' requests for more clinical and practical information. *Seminars in Oncology Nursing*, a quarterly journal presenting comprehensive coverage within topical reviews, began publication in 1984. The *European Journal of Oncology Nursing*, the official journal of the European Oncology Nursing Society (EONS), began publication in 1996.

Creation and dissemination of standards of oncology nursing care

The influence of the ONS on cancer nursing is undeniable. Its growth, member services, and diverse projects and programming reflect the needs and interests of cancer nurses worldwide. From its 226 charter members in 1975, the ONS membership in 2008 includes approximately 35,000 members. Nearly 40% of those members also claim membership in at least one of 220 local chapters, allowing for rapid dissemination of information relevant to members and maintenance of local and regional exchange of information and resources. In the early history of ONS, local chapter members were involved in drafting standards of care, and in 1979 the ONS and the American Nurses Association published *Outcome Standards for Cancer Nursing Practice* [63]. The *Statement on the Scope and Standards of Oncology Nursing Practice* [64] followed in 1987, and the initial *Standards of Advanced Practice in Oncology Nursing* [65] was issued in 1990. These and subsequent documents represent expert oncology nursing consensus of desired outcomes with regard to physical, psychosocial, and spiritual aspects of cancer care.

Support for subspecialties

Special Interest Groups (SIGs) were established as a formal organizational component of the ONS in 1989. Eighteen SIGs were chartered that year; in 2007, 29 SIGs allow members to network, communicate, and play roles in the evolution of subspecialty interests. (Complete ONS SIG information can be obtained at the ONS Web site: Ref. [66]).

Global impact

The ONS has been a catalyst for national and regional oncology nursing organizations throughout the world. The EONS was incorporated in 1984 and now has individual and organizational members [67]. The International Society of Nurses in Cancer Care, also incorporated in 1984, is an international network offering support and communication for national and regional cancer nursing societies. The International Union Against Cancer supports an active nursing committee, with delegates from several nations, responsible for planning and delivering cancer nursing education in developing countries.

Policy and politics

Today's cancer nurses are cognizant of the impact of policy and politics on their own nursing practice and their various practice settings. Still, the majority of nurses, including cancer nurses, remain outside or on the fringes of health care's political arena and the profession continues to be an untapped political resource [68]. Many policy and political issues are of importance to nurses in general but take on special significance in cancer care; among them are ways to address the nursing shortage, measures to optimize the use of advance practice nurses, responses to the epidemic of errors in health care settings, care of the nation's older people, strategies to reform the United States health care system, access to care and the growing population of uninsured, and measures to address the health needs of diverse populations. Many policy issues are of particular interest to cancer nurses and other cancer care providers. For example, the National Institutes of

Health estimate overall costs of cancer exceed $200 billion annually [69]. Hematopoietic growth factors, commonly used in myelosuppressive therapy regimens, are Medicare's single largest expenditure, exceeding $10 billion in 2006 [70].

The goal of increasing and enhancing cancer nurses' roles in the political arena has yet to be achieved. Evidence demonstrative of nurses' minimal influence is clear when reviewing nursing representation—or lack thereof—in policy-setting initiatives. Three reports released between 2006 and 2007 by the Institute of Medicine were prepared by committees, each with one nurse in multidisciplinary groups of between 10 and 20 members composed primarily of physicians [71–73]. None of these reports, which often are cited in policy-making circles, accurately reflects the importance of nurses' ongoing work in these settings nor do they provide support for nurses' future roles in addressing these relevant social and health issues. Likewise, payment for cancer care planning, described in the Comprehensive Cancer Care Improvement Act of 2007, is categorized under Medicare's physician fee schedule, minimizing contributions to these efforts by nurses, social workers, and other disciplines [74]. These examples provide evidence that oncology nurses have yet to achieve a preferred level of substantive roles in policy-making arenas.

The future of cancer nursing

The future of cancer nursing will derive from the actions of today's cancer nursing leaders. For more than 2 decades, nurse leaders have expressed pessimism about the future outlook for their profession, pondering what the future holds given the disorienting turbulence created by the massive changes occurring in health care around the world and the paucity of leaders prepared and willing to plan and effect necessary changes [75,76]. The magic bullet, the treatment regimen that will cure cancers once and for all, has not been discovered and is unlikely to be any time soon. An aging population, high-risk health behaviors, environmental pollutants, and infectious diseases contribute to development of cancer, assuring the ongoing need for cancer nursing. Kitson [76] suggests that future-directed strategies must be

> ...built upon a unity of purpose and a shared vision, not just within nursing but also shared with medical colleagues, chief executives, politicians, and the public. Nursing in the future needs to be seen as part of the solution rather than contributing to the problem. Nursing, as one of health care's solutions, will indeed herald an exciting future and one which we must ensure is valued and promoted.

New normal for cancer nurses

Advances in technology and science have given rise to at least four new populations of concern to cancer care providers: individuals at increased risk for development of cancer; individuals who are living with cancer as a chronic disease; individuals who live with advanced and metastatic disease; and long-term survivors. The existence of these populations is, in large part, a goal that cancer care providers have pursued for decades. Now that people survive primary therapy, it is clear that there has been failure to plan for the needs that occur in the emerging phases of the cancer experience [77]. As the survivorship experience progresses, disease-oriented physicians have less to offer whereas health-oriented care providers, such as nurses, social workers, nutritionists, rehabilitation specialists, psychologists, and physicians who do adapt to more health-oriented contributions, assume greater significance in the lives of long-term survivors [78,79]. For these providers to perform optimally, the medicalization of cancer care must end and a more patient-centered team approach must be crafted and nurtured [80]. Cancer survivors are advised to find and value the "new normal" in their lives after cancer [81]. Nurses and other cancer care providers need to heed the same advice, integrating emerging realities into a new normal of cancer care delivery.

Integration of caring, science, and technology

The evolution of cancer diagnostics and therapies continues at an unprecedented rate. The application and success of technologies introduced into patient care are, for the most part, dependent on nurses [82]. It generally is nurses who connect machines to persons, assume competencies associated with new technology, calm fears generated by machines, and humanize the technology-driven experience [82,83]. The critical nature of patients who have cancer in contemporary and future acute, community, and home care settings makes it likely that technologic devices, including life-system support and monitors, fluid and medication delivery systems, electronic assessment tools, and electronic data banks, will be used at the bedside, chairside, and in homes. Nurses who offer wise guidance in clients' adoption of health behaviors and patients' treatment decision making offer care and assistance at crucial times throughout the cancer trajectory. Nurses involved in the care of people concerned about or directly affected by cancer must be knowledgeable about scientific advances, including those in the research pipeline, to anticipate and meet the informational and nursing care needs of the populations being served. Scientific advances offer the potential to determine, with more accuracy, individuals' risk for developing cancer and the risks and benefits associated with various treatment options. Next-generation cancer therapies, including more selective use of chemotherapy, oral and self-administration of chemotherapy, availability of more targeted therapies, biologics, vaccines, gene therapy, and proton therapy, are associated with unknown, new, or different side-effect and toxicity profiles that cancer nurses need to understand and include in routine teaching, guidance, facilitation of treatment adherence, and caring for patients, family, and other caregivers [84].

Information technology

Next-generation nurses will of necessity be not only computer literate but also skilled in the creation, access, use, and sharing of electronically generated data and information. There is a slow but steady movement toward implementation of electronic medical records, something Henderson [85] considered more than 2 decades ago. She believed patient-held medical information is a means of empowering patients—and a way for nurses to develop more equal partnerships with patients [85]. The long-term nature of cancer care makes it imperative that patients and clients have and maintain information about their diagnoses, treatment, plans for medical follow-up, and guidance for life-long healthy lifestyles, as recommended in the Institute of Medicine's report, *From Cancer Patient to Cancer Survivor* [71]. Nurses can be critical in the creation of user-friendly tools and documents that serve the needs of providers and patients, families, and clients [84,86].

The vast amount of information available to the public requires interpretation, giving nurses opportunities as knowledge brokers for every patient and client. Nurses can be involved in helping patients and clients access and understand information, provideing information about specialists, resources, and complementary and alternative modalities. Nurses need highly developed assessment, listening, communication, and teaching skills and clear understanding of patients' and clients' values and ethical principles to guide choices and informed decision making.

Nurses must be involved in creation of mechanisms to assure clients' health information is used appropriately. The efficacy and impact—positive and negative—of computer-based educational materials, decision aids, and direct-to-consumer marketing will be dependent on the kind of human interactions that nurses can provide.

Presence

Cancer nurses of the future must be positioned, available, visible, and present wherever there are actual and potential patients and clients. Illness care settings largely have shifted back to communities, with care occurring increasingly in physician offices, community ambulatory clinics, and homes, whereas acute patient care needs are increasingly critical and intense [87,88]. Wellness-oriented care, too, occurs in community settings [88]. Nurses' community-level contributions will be increasingly important and the emphasis of nurses' education likewise must shift from acute care to community settings [89]. It is equally important that nurses provide quality health care features consistent with patients' needs, values, and preferences [90]. The shift in cancer care settings requires new appraisals of nursing roles, preparation, and competencies [88–92].

Policy issues created by this shift are complex and unresolved. Adequate staffing, roles, competencies, and desired outcomes have yet to be defined for the diverse cancer care settings [87,90,91]. The dispute over practice expense and drug reimbursement focuses on the way the Centers for Medicare and Medicaid Services (CMS) value services rendered in offices by nonphysicians [93]. Under the current Medicare system, outpatient oncology nursing services are classified and paid for as a practice expense with little consideration of the nursing expertise, knowledge, skill levels, and relative autonomy inherent in nursing practice in these settings.

The public, the discipline's greatest ally in assuring the survival of nursing as a viable profession, must know who nurses are and what care they provide [94]. More than a decade ago, nurses were described as "health care's invisible partner" in *The Woodhull Study on Nursing and the Media* [95], a situation that contributes to nursing work being discounted in policy-making agendas. There has been no formal follow-up to *The Woodhull Study*, and whether or not nursing is more visible since 1997 is unclear, but there is ample evidence that the contributions of nursing remain undervalued. As an example, research presented at oncology conferences targeting physicians regularly makes the evening television news and the morning newspapers: there is little or no coverage of conferences presenting cancer-related clinical nursing innovations or nursing research. Nurses must make sure they are visible to those on the "receiving end of our care"—people who can write letters to payers and policy makers or who may be health care administrators, board members, and local and national government officials [94]. Activities performed by nurses, outcomes, and how they are classified for potential payment, particularly in office-based settings, must be explored. To date, only the American Society of Clinical Oncology has explored and submitted practice expense data, including the nursing component, to CMS [96]. Nurses, not physicians or policy makers, must do this.

Support for the cancer nursing workforce

If nurses are to be present and available to persons facing cancer, the adequacy, competencies, and general welfare of the cancer nursing workforce must be assured. The quality and quantity of cancer care are expected to fall short of demands because of supply limitations of medical and radiation oncologists, oncology nurses, social workers, and other professional providers that are becoming apparent [97]. C-Change is a nonprofit collaboration of the public, private, and nonprofit sectors to address cancer-related issues and challenges, including expanding the cancer care workforce [97,98]. The ONS, American Society of Clinical Oncology, National Association of Social Workers, and American Society for Therapeutic and Radiation Oncology are among the 130 C-Change participants [98]. An initial C-Change goal involves building a National Cancer Corps, strengthening the knowledge and skills of the nononcology health workforce, with a surge capacity designed to meet the more immediate needs of the aging and diverse American population [97,98].

Attention must be given to initial recruitment of young people into the nursing profession, beginning with understanding the personal and career motivations of the new generation of potential nurses—variously called generation Y, millennium generation, and echo-boomer generation—the demographic cohort born after 1981 [99]. Members of the generation Y cohort are described as materialistic, disrespectful, technologically literate, and as having a pragmatic worldview. Career choices among members of generation Y seem driven by their desire for meaningful roles in work that helps others, and they feel comfortable moving quickly among jobs to find a good fit [99]. Integration of identified generational career motivation factors must be integrated with current and future nursing student recruitment and workforce retention strategies.

There is no end in sight to the current nursing shortage, and nursing leaders need to pursue creative strategies to recruit and retain, using nurses' education, expertise, and experience most effectively. An unknown but increasing number of nurses is pursuing non-nursing advanced degrees. Nurses holding master's and doctoral degrees in business administration, education, psychology, physiology, thanatology, medical ethics, and public health (to list a few of many advanced study areas selected by nurses) often follow nontraditional career courses, many of them employed in non-nursing occupations. In the 2004 National Sample Survey of Registered Nurses, 14% (nearly one-half million) of registered nurses were not working in nursing; nearly half of those had left nursing for personal, career, and workplace reasons [100]. The viability and vitality of nursing will be enhanced when the experience and expertise of these nurses is valued, embraced, and applied to nursing education, practice, research, and management.

Cancer nurses are at high risk for work-related stress relating to chronic compounded grief, exposure to patients' and families' suffering, frequent crises, emotional experiences, and death among a high percentage of people in their care [101]. Such stressors are complicated by a health care environment characterized by nursing shortages, diminishing levels of supportive personnel, limited budgets, paperwork demands, and complex therapies and technologies. The consequences of unrelieved job stress include compassion fatigue and burnout among nurses with associated negative effects on quality of care, patient and nurse work satisfaction, nurse recruitment, retention issues and job turnover costs, and morbidity among nurses [102,103]. Increasing management and research attention must be given to practice setting characteristics, including effective communication, minimization of workplace conflict, high levels of nurse autonomy, manageable workload, and support from supervisors and coworkers, that diminish risks for compassion fatigue among cancer nurses [101–103]. Every nurse, regardless of practice setting, can learn and use appropriate self-care skills and help create and maintain a supportive and healthy workplace environment; workforce managers must provide leadership, flexibility, and opportunities that foster a healthy workplace.

Patient/client navigation

Despite scientific advances in cancer care, some populations, most notably the poor and underserved, bear a disproportionate burden of cancer, with higher incidence and mortality and lower survival rates [104]. Many challenges are associated with the aging population, including greater disabilities after cancer treatment and the likelihood of diminished personal and fiscal resources [105]. Health disparities pose challenges for the cancer care community and continue to be among America's most difficult moral and ethical dilemmas. In an effort to break down economic, social, and cultural barriers, a model Patient Navigation Program using trained lay navigators was initiated at Harlem Hospital Center in New York City [106]. Although the model program was based on the hospital's breast cancer experience, evaluative data showed improvements in disease stage at diagnosis and 5-year survival rates, suggesting that patient navigation programs could be applied to all cancers [106]. The concept of patient navigation was given further support during ongoing town hall meetings of the President's Cancer Panel in the years 2000 and 2001, resulting in the Panel's recommendation of increased public funding to help communities coordinate, promote, and support community-based programs to help people get cancer information, screening, treatment, and supportive services [105]. The Patient Navigator Act of 2005 (Pub.L.No.109-018) established a patient navigator demonstration program through the Health Resources Services Administration (HRSA) linked to activities at the NCI [107].

Concerns have been expressed that initial legislative language failed to stipulate supervision and oversight of lay navigators by licensed professionals. The National Association of Social Workers is among several stakeholder groups working to develop guidelines to help HRSA and the NCI in the demonstration projects [107]. Oncology nurses and oncology social workers are assuming patient navigator roles, called navigators, case managers, coaches, or other titles, with varying role expectations [108–110]. A C-Change workgroup prepared a useful definition of patient navigation that does not specify underlying credentials but instead focuses on expectations and outcomes [111]:

> Patient navigation in cancer care refers to individualized assistance offered to patients, families, and caregivers to help overcome health care system barriers and facilitate timely access to quality medical and psychosocial care from pre-diagnosis through all phases of the cancer experience. Navigation services and programs should be provided by culturally competent professional or non-professional persons in a variety of medical, organizational, advocacy, or community settings. The type of navigation services will depend upon the particular type, severity, and/or complexity of the identified barriers.

Broad knowledge about all aspects of health care that nurses can provide is a priceless resource for helping people make decisions about their health and offers competencies for patient navigation services. Regardless of title or professional or lay preparation, navigation goals should remain those proposed by the President's Cancer Panel [105]:

- No person who has cancer should go untreated.
- No person who has cancer should be bankrupted by a diagnosis of cancer.
- No person who has cancer should be forced to spend more time fighting his or her way through the health care system than fighting his or her disease.

Although enthusiasm for separate and distinct patient navigation roles is apparent, adapting existing advanced nursing practice competencies might be considered, in particular those traditionally attributed to oncology clinical nurse specialist roles (clinician, consultant, educator, change agent, and researcher) [112] to meet needs identified as rationale for patient navigators. The notion of a community oncology nurse specialist has been explored in the United Kingdom and found to be a potentially valuable role [113]. Kaiser and colleagues [114] described outcomes and competencies to guide curriculum changes necessary for advanced practice community or public health nurses, who could meet needs similar to those underlying patient navigator roles. Given the reality of patients and clients increasingly receiving care in community settings, it is logical to reconsider the education and competencies of general and advanced practice nurses to meet the evolving needs associated with contemporary and future cancer care [115].

Summary

The contemporary domain of cancer nursing has an undeniably long and rich history. The nursing of people who have cancer predates scientific and technologic innovations that made control or cure achievable for a majority of people affected by the disease. Cancer nurses and the people they serve are beneficiaries of the vision, passion, commitment, and guidance of generations of nurses who preceded them. Past and present cancer nursing leaders and the millions of overlooked others share a belief that the status quo of their circumstances is unacceptable and shared the wisdom, passion, and commitment to create meaningful change. A desire to make a difference for people facing the challenges of cancer has been and remains the essence of cancer nursing [116]. The circumstances of patients, clients, families, communities, and nurses of 2008 have improved immeasurably: overall cancer survival rates now are close to 70% and symptom management strategies are not only possible but also accepted standard practice. Yet, the status quo in many aspects of cancer care is unacceptable. For cancer nurses, some things remain remarkably unchanged, as revealed in the foreword of *A Cancer Source Book for Nurses* released more than 4 decades ago:

It may be that no other disease demands of the nurse so much sympathetic understanding of human relationships as well as knowledge of the disease itself. Probably no other illness requires such wise guidance in building morale to help the patient and his family meet their problems [117].

References

[1] Johnson J, editor. Those were hard days [videotape]. Pittsburgh (PA): Oncology Nursing Society; 1985.

[2] Scovil ER. Notes from the medical Press. Am J Nurs 1913;13:780–2.

[3] Yarbro CH. The history of cancer nursing. In: Baird SB, McCorkle R, Grant M, editors. Cancer nursing: a comprehensive textbook. Philadelphia: W.B. Saunders; 1991. p. 10–20.

[4] Nevidjon B, editor. Building a legacy: voices of oncology nurses. Boston: Jones & Bartlett; 1995.

[5] Haylock PJ. Virginia Barckley. In: Bullough VL, Sentz L, editors. American nursing: a biographical dictionary, vol. 3. New York: Springer Publishing; 2000. p. 14–6.

[6] Dudas S, Renilda E. Hilkemeyer. In: Bullough VL, Sentz L, editors. American nursing: a biographical dictionary, vol. 3. New York: Springer Publishing Company; 2000. p. 137–40.

[7] Johnson J, Baird S, Hilderley L, editors. It took courage, compassion, and curiosity: recollections and writings of leaders in cancer nursing: 1890–1970. Pittsburgh (PA): Oncology Nursing Society Publishing Division; 2001.

[8] Hilkemeyer R. Oral history. Pittsburgh (PA): Located at Oncology Nursing Society Archives; 1995.

[9] Lusk B. Overlooked solders in the cancer wars: nurses and cancer, 1880–1950. Available at: http://archive.rockefeller.edu/publications/resrep/lusk.pdf. Accessed November 21, 2007.

[10] Lusk B. Prelude to specialization: US cancer nursing, 1920–1950. Nurs Inq 2005;12:269–77.

[11] First cancer nursing course. The New York Times. July 3, 1944.

[12] Nixon RM. Acting against cancer. The Saturday Evening Post. July/August 1986;258: 67–9.

[13] Shimkin MB. Contrary to nature. Washington, DC: U.S. Government Printing Office; 1977, DHEW Publication No. [NIH] 76-720.

[14] Yarbro JW. Milestones in our understanding of cancer. In: Groenwald SL, Frogge MH, Goodman M, et al, editors. Cancer nursing principles and practice. 4th edition. Boston: Jones & Bartlett; 1997. p. 3–16.

[15] Minkowski WL. Women healers of the middle ages: selected aspects of their history. Am J Public Health 1992;82:288–95.

[16] Sparkman RS. Presidential address: the woman in the case—Jane Todd Crawford, 1763–1842. Ann Surg 1979;189:529–45.

[17] Agnew JW. Abdomino-perineal resection. Am J Nurs 1951;51:225–6.

[18] Strueben EM. Nursing care for the patient with an abdomino-perineal resection. Am J Nurs 1951;51:226–8.

[19] Hilkemeyer R. A historical perspective in cancer nursing. Oncol Nurs Forum 1985; 12(Suppl 1):6–15.

[20] The etiology of cancer. JAMA 1898;30:1119.

[21] The transmission and care of cancer. Am J Nurs 1907;8:200.

[22] Levin I. The cancer problem and the nurse. Am J Nurs 1927;27:83–9.

[23] Ashley J. Hospitals, paternalism, and the role of the nurse. New York: Teachers College Press; 1976.

[24] Buhler-Wilkerson K. No place like home: a history of nursing and home care in the United States. Baltimore (MD): The Johns Hopkins Press; 2001.

[25] Starr P. The social transformation of American medicine. (USA): Basic Books; 1982.

[26] Stern G. Sainthood proposed for Rose Lathrop of Hawthorne. The Journal News. February 5, 2003. Available at: http://home.sprynet.com/~rblathrop/genealogy/rose_hawthorne_lathrop_05201851.htm. Accessed November 18, 2007.
[27] Maynard T. A fire was lighted. Milwaukee (WI): Bruce Publishing Company; 1948.
[28] Valenti PD. To myself a stranger: a biography of Rose Hawthorne Lathrop. Baton Rouge (LA): Louisiana State University Press; 1991.
[29] Drown LL. Progressive movements: a successful experiment. Am J Nurs 1901;1:729–31.
[30] Sleet JC. A successful experiment. Am J Nurs 1901;1:729–31.
[31] Link G. Modern gynaecology: an address before the Indiana State Nurses' Association. Am J Nurs 1911;11:266–70.
[32] Gilman AS. The eight-hour day for the three hundred-bed hospital. Am J Nurs 1919;19: 294–6.
[33] Barckley V. The best of times and the worst of times: historical reflections from an American Cancer Society National Nursing Consultant. Oncol Nurs Forum 1985;12(Suppl 1): 16–8.
[34] Kelly J. Some psychological aspects of gynecological nursing. Am J Nurs 1938;3:470–2.
[35] Ferris AA. The nursing care of cancer patients: some recent developments. Am J Nurs 1930; 30:814–20.
[36] Berdjis CC. Pathology of irradiation. Baltimore (MD): Williams and Wilkins Co; 1971.
[37] Gibson AL. Radium, radon, radiumtherapy. Am J Nurs 1930;30:967–74.
[38] Burke MB, Wilkes GM, Berg D, et al, editors. Cancer chemotherapy and nursing practice: a unique blend. Cancer chemotherapy: a nursing process approach. Boston: Jones & Bartlett; 1996. p. 3–14.
[39] Zubrod CG. Historic milestones in curative chemotherapy. Semin Oncol 1979;6:490–505.
[40] Nelson K. The history of cancer in the nursing curriculum, 1860–1951. In: Proceedings: cancer nurses make it happen: a tenth anniversary history of the nursing committee. Wallingford (CT): American Cancer Society, Connecticut Division; 1987.
[41] Joint Committee of the National Organization for Public Health Nursing and the United States Public Health Service. The public health nurse curriculum guide. 1942.
[42] Johnson V. The nursing care of patients with carcinoma. Am J Nurs 1934;34:768–71.
[43] Best N. Radiotherapy and the nurse. Am J Nurs 1950;50:140–3.
[44] Kendall S. Being asked not to tell: nurses' experiences of caring for cancer patients not told their diagnosis. J Clin Nurs 2006;15:1149–57.
[45] Barckley V. The crises in cancer. Am J Nurs 1967;67:278–80.
[46] Barckley V. What can I say to the cancer patient? Nurs Outlook 1958;6:316–8.
[47] Hopp M. Roentgen therapy and the nurse. Am J Nurs 1941;41:431–3.
[48] Glienke F, Kress LC. The cancer patient: planning for and introducing home care. Am J Nurs 1944;44:351–4.
[49] Glienke F, Kress LC. The cancer patient: giving bedside care in the home. Am J Nurs 1944; 44:434–43.
[50] Hirsch J. An anniversary for cancer chemotherapy. JAMA 2006;296:1518–20.
[51] Hilkemeyer R, Kinney HE. Teaching cancer nursing. Nurs Outlook 1956;4:177–80.
[52] Peterson RI. Knowledge of cancer—equipment for nursing. Am J Nurs 1954;54:463–6.
[53] Golbey RB. Chemotherapy of cancer. Am J Nurs 1960;60:521–5.
[54] Ferris AA. Fifty grams of radium. Am J Nurs 1953;53:1080–1.
[55] American Cancer Society. A cancer source book for nurses. New York: American Cancer Society; 1950.
[56] National Cancer Institute, United States Public Health Service, and the New York State Department of Health. Cancer nursing: a manual for public health nurses. Bethesda (MD): National Cancer Institute; 1950.
[57] Handorf LL, Pedersen TE. Nursing care in terminal cancer. Am J Nurs 1950;50:643–6.
[58] Lynaugh JE. Nursing the great society: the impact of the Nurse Training Act of 1964. Nurs Hist Rev 2008;16:13–28.

[59] Hubbard SM, Donehower MG. The nurse in a cancer research setting. Semin Oncol 1980;7: 9–17.
[60] Henke C. Emerging roles of the nurse in oncology. Semin Oncol 1980;7:4–8.
[61] Ash CR. The past...the present...the future.... Cancer Nurs 2007;30:419.
[62] Greene PE. The Association of Pediatric Oncology Nurses: the first ten years. Oncol Nurs Forum 1985;12(Suppl):44–8.
[63] American Nurses Association and Oncology Nursing Society. Outcome standards of cancer nursing practice. Washington, DC: American Nurses Association; 1979.
[64] Oncology Nursing Society. Statement on the scope and standards of oncology nursing practice. Pittsburgh (PA): Oncology Nursing Society; 1987.
[65] Oncology Nursing Society. Standards of advanced practice in oncology nursing. Pittsburgh (PA): Oncology Nursing Society; 1990.
[66] ONS Membership SIG List. Available at: http://www.ons.org. Accessed March 30, 2008.
[67] European Oncology Nursing Society. President's report: November 2005–September 2007. Available at: http://www.cancerworld.org/CancerWorld/getStaticModFile.aspx?id=1944. Accessed December 20, 2007.
[68] Mason DJ, Levitt JK, Chaffee MW. Policy and politics in nursing and health care. 5th edition. St. Louis (MO): Saunders; 2007.
[69] American Cancer Society. Cancer facts & figures 2007. Available at: http://www.cancer.org/downloads/STT/CAFF2007PWSecured.pdf. Accessed December 18, 2007.
[70] Steinbrook R. Erythropoietin, the FDA, and oncology. N Engl J Med 2007;356:2448–51.
[71] Hewitt M, Greenfield S, Stovall E, editors. From cancer patient to cancer survivor: lost in transition. Washington, DC: National Academies Press; 2006 [Institute of Medicine and National Research Council].
[72] Sloan FA, Gelband H. Cancer control opportunities in low- and middle-income countries. Washington, DC: National Academies Press; 2007.
[73] Institute of Medicine. Cancer care for the whole patient: meeting psychosocial health needs. Washington, DC: National Academies Press; 2007.
[74] The Comprehensive Cancer Care Improvement Act of 2007. 110th Congress. Available at: http://thomas.loc.gov/home/gpoxmlc110/h1078_ih.xml. Accessed December 20, 2007.
[75] Schlotfeldt RM. A brave, new nursing world: exercising options for the future. Washington, DC: American Association of Colleges of Nursing; 1982. Publication Series 82, No. 3.
[76] Kitson AL. Johns Hopkins address: does nursing have a future? Image J Nurs Sch 1997;29: 111–5.
[77] Earle CC. Failing to plan is planning to fail: improving the quality of care with survivorship care plans. J Clin Oncol 2006;24:5112–6.
[78] Kramberg L. Quality care for cancer survivors: the case for comprehensive cancer care. Silver Spring (MD): A White Paper for the National Coalition for Cancer Survivorship; 2005.
[79] Feuerstein M, Findley P. The cancer survivor's guide: the essential handbook to life after cancer. New York: Marlowe and Company; 2006.
[80] Hall B. An essay on an authentic meaning of medicalization. ANS Adv Nurs Sci 2003;26: 53–62.
[81] Harpham WS. Happiness in a storm: facing illness and embracing life as a healthy survivor. New York: WW Norton & Co; 2005. p. 17.
[82] Fairman J. Alternative visions: the nurse-technology relationship in the context of the history of technology. Nurs Hist Rev 1998;6:129–46.
[83] McConnell EA. The coalescence of technology and humansism in nursing practice: it doesn't just happen and it doesn't come easily. Holist Nurs Pract 1998;12(4):23–30.
[84] Moore S. Facilitating oral chemotherapy treatment and compliance through patient/family-focused education. Cancer Nurs 2007;30:112–22.
[85] Henderson VA. The essence of nursing in high technology. Nurs Adm Q 1985;9(4):1–9.

[86] Haylock PJ, Mitchell SA, Cox T, et al. The cancer survivors' prescription for living. Am J Nurs 2007;107(4):58–70.

[87] Ireland AM, DePalma JA, Arneson L, et al. The Oncology Nursing Society ambulatory office nurse survey. Oncol Nurs Forum 2004;31:E147–56.

[88] Vlasses FR, Smeltzer CH. Toward a new future for healthcare and nursing practice. J Nurs Adm 2007;37:375–80.

[89] Schim SM, Thornburg P, Kravutske ME. Time, task, and talents in ambulatory care nursing. J Nurs Adm 2001;31:311–5.

[90] Jennings BM, Hemman EA, Heiner SL, et al. What really matters to healthcare consumers. J Nurs Adm 2005;35:173–80.

[91] Levac K. Putting outcomes into practice in physician offices. J Nurs Care Qual 2002;17: 51–62.

[92] Thompson P, Lulham K. Clinical nurse leader and clinical nurse specialist role delineation in the acute care setting. J Nurs Adm 2007;37:429–31.

[93] Iglehart JK. Medicare and drug pricing. N Engl J Med 2003;348:1590–7.

[94] Tulman L. Phantom nurses are real bedsides. Nurs Outlook 1997;45:239.

[95] Sigma Theta Tau, International. The Woodhull study on nursing and the media: health care's invisible partner. Indianpolis (IN): Center Nursing Press, Sigma Theta Tau International; 2007.

[96] Dobson A, Koenig L, Siegel J, et al. The Lewin Group. Recommendations regarding supplemental practice expense data submitted for 2003: evaluation of survey data for: physical therapy, oncology, cardiology, pediatrics. Prepared for Centers for Medicare and Medicaid Services, #500-95-0059/TO#6. September 17, 2002.

[97] Smith AP, Lichtveld MY. A competency-based approach to expanding the cancer care workforce. Nurs Econ 2007;25:110–8.

[98] C-Change. About C-Change. Available at: http://www.c-changetogether.org/about_ndc/default.asp. Accessed December 16, 2007.

[99] Sadler JJ. Who wants to be a nurse: motivation of the new generation. J Prof Nurs 2003;19: 173–5.

[100] Department of Health and Human Services, Health Resources and Services Administration Bureau of Health Professions. The registered nurse population: findings from the March 2004 national sample survey of registered nurses. 2006. Available at: http://ftp://ftp.hrsa.gov/bhpr/workforce/0306 rnss.pdf. Accessed December 26, 2007.

[101] Medland J, Howard-Ruben J, Whitaker E. Fostering psychosocial wellness in oncology nurses: addressing burnout and social support in the workplace. Oncol Nurs Forum 2004;31:47–54.

[102] Sabo BM. Compassion fatigue and nursing work: can we accurately capture the consequences of caring work? Int J Nurs Pract 2006;12:136–42.

[103] Cohen-Katz J, Wiley SD, Capuano T, et al. The effects of mindfulness-based stress reduction on nurse stress and burnout: a quantitative and qualitative study. Holist Nurs Pract 2004;18:302–8.

[104] Haynes MA, Smedley BD, editors. The unequal burden of cancer: an Assessment of National Institute of Health Research and Programs for Ethnic Minorities and the Medically Underserved. Washington, DC: National Academies Press; 1999. [Institute of Medicine].

[105] President's Cancer Panel. Chairman. Voices of a broken system: real people, real problems 2000–2001. Bethesda (MD): National Cancer Institute; 2001.

[106] Freeman HP. A model patient navigation program. Oncol Issues 2004;6:44–6.

[107] National Association of Social Workers. Office of Government Relations and Political Action. January-March 2006. Patient Navigator Act. Available at: http://www.socialworkers.org/advocacy/updates/2006/GRLEGagendaopt2006_0103.pdf. Accessed December 18, 2007.

[108] Schwaderer KA, Itano JK. Bridging the healthcare divide with patient navigation: development of a research program to address disparities. Clin J Oncol Nurs 2007;11: 633–9.
[109] Canadian Breast Cancer Initiative. Investigation and Assessment of the Navigator Role in Meeting the Information, Decisional and Educational Needs of Women with Breast Cancer in Canada. Her Majesty the Queen in Right of Canada, represented by the Minister of Public Works and Government Services Canada. Cat. N̊ H39–663/2002E, ISBN 0-662-33232; 2001.
[110] Bruce S. Taking the wheel: oncology nurses help patients navigate the cancer journey. ONS Connect 2007;2(3):8–11.
[111] C-Change: patient navigator. Available at: http://www.cancerpatientnavigation.org/navigation/other_resources.html. Accessed December 16, 2007.
[112] Spross J. An overview of the oncology clinical nurse specialist role. Oncol Nurs Forum 1983;10(3):54–8.
[113] Vooght S, Richardson A. A study to explore the role of a community oncology nurse specialist. Eur J Cancer Care 1996;5:217–24.
[114] Kaiser KL, Barr KL, Hays BJ. Setting a new course for advanced practice community/public health nursing. J Prof Nurs 2003;19:189–96.
[115] Hamric AB, Hanson CM. Educating advanced practice nurses for practice reality. J Prof Nurs 2003;19:262–8.
[116] Steeves R, Cohen MZ, Wise CT. An analysis of critical incidents describing the essence of oncology nursing. Oncol Nurs Forum 1994;21(Suppl 8):19–25.
[117] American Cancer Society, Inc. A cancer source book for nurses. New York: American Cancer Society; 1963.

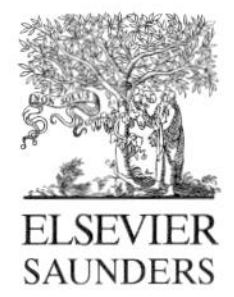

ELSEVIER
SAUNDERS

Nurs Clin N Am 43 (2008) 205–220

NURSING
CLINICS
OF NORTH AMERICA

Symptom Management Issues in Oncology Nursing

Lisa Schulmeister, RN, MN, APRN-BC, OCN, FAAN[a,*], Barbara Holmes Gobel, RN, MS, AOCN[b,c]

[a]*282 Orchard Road, River Ridge, LA 70123-2648, USA*
[b]*Northwestern Memorial Hospital, 251 East Huron-Feinberg Pavilion 4-508, Chicago, IL 60011, USA*
[c]*5400 Grand Avenue, Western Springs, IL 60558-1840, USA*

Symptoms experienced by patients with cancer can occur as a direct effect of the disease process and be related to side effects of treatment. Many patients with cancer also are older in age and have comorbidities, such as diabetes and heart disease. Comorbid conditions also produce disease and treatment-related symptoms that may have an independent or compounding effect on cancer-related symptoms.

Until recently, oncology nurses tended to focus on one symptom at a time. When a patient reported pain, pain intensity was assessed (usually on a 0–10 scale) and managed accordingly. Currently there is increased recognition that symptoms often occur together, or cluster [1]. Nurses assess for additional symptoms when pain is reported because evidence suggests that pain clusters with other symptoms, such as fatigue, sleep disturbance, depression, and anorexia [2,3]. Identifying symptoms that cluster may aid in identifying ways to better manage symptoms. Evidenced-based symptom management has the potential to improve patient outcomes, promote patient and nurse satisfaction, and reduce costs to the health care system [4].

Symptom measurement

Symptoms are subjective experiences that evolve and change over time. Each patient's treatment experience is unique, and the patient's symptom experience is influenced in large part by how a patient responds to treatment of cancer and other diseases or conditions [5]. Symptom measurement may

* Corresponding author.
E-mail address: lisaschulmeister@hotmail.com (L. Schulmeister).

0029-6465/08/$ - see front matter
doi:10.1016/j.cnur.2008.02.004

be complicated or influenced by several factors. Cultural influences impact how patients perceive, report, and cope with symptoms. For instance, patients may believe that adverse symptoms are to be expected as part of the cancer experience. Language barriers may impair symptom assessment and measurement. Patients may be unable to report symptoms because of coma, cognitive impairment, or other conditions. Measurement of symptoms experienced by children, especially very young children, is challenging [6–8].

Kirkova and colleagues [9] conducted a systematic review of cancer symptom assessment instruments. They identified 21 instruments that were purported to measure cancer symptoms and located 28 additional studies that used some of the instruments to examine symptom interrelations or clusters. The instruments varied in the number and type of symptoms measured, and many lacked psychometric testing and validation. The symptoms of pain, fatigue, and anorexia were included in all of the instruments that measured five or more symptoms. Sixteen of the instruments were designed for general use in oncology, and 5 were specific to measuring cancer treatment-related effects, such as chemotherapy-induced nausea and vomiting. Comprehensive instruments that were deemed acceptable for use in clinical and research settings and found to have acceptable psychometric properties are listed in Fig. 1. The researchers did not find any instrument that met all of their criteria for an ideal instrument (eg, has comprehensive content, assesses symptom clusters, is easy to understand and complete, is reliable and accurate, discriminates, and facilitates initial and ongoing symptom control). Prospective controlled clinical trials are needed to compare validated instruments and identify the best instruments to use in clinical practice. Findings from these clinical trials also may guide the development of guidelines for comprehensive cancer symptom measurement and management [9].

Symptom clusters

The term "symptom cluster" has been defined in various ways. The common thread among the definitions is that a system cluster is composed of two or more symptoms that are related to each other and occur together [10,11]. Symptom clusters are composed of stable groups of symptoms, are relatively independent of other symptom clusters, and may share the same origin or have different origins [12]. Relationships between and among the symptoms may be complex [13].

There are two main approaches to identifying symptom clusters. Clusters may be clinically identified and statistically analyzed for association (or lack of association) among the symptoms. These predefined clusters generally have five or fewer symptoms, and examples of symptom clusters identified using this approach include the cluster of pain, fatigue, and insomnia and the cluster of pain, depression, and fatigue. Symptom clusters also may be

Computerized Symptom Assessment Instrument

The instrument contains 20 core items on a bar-type scale that assess physical, psychological, and functional domains, presence, and symptom distress. There are additional item sets specific to breast, lung, and head and neck cancer. The instrument is completed by the patient.

Memorial Symptom Assessment Scale (MSAS)

The scale contains 32 Likert type items that assess physical and psychosocial domains and calculate a global distress index score. Frequency, severity, and symptom distress are measured and the scale is completed by the patient.

Oncology Treatment Toxicity Scale (OTTAT)

The scale contains 37 Likert type items that assess physical, psychosocial, and functional domains and includes items that assess symptom frequency and severity. A summated score is calculated and the scale is completed by the patient.

Rotterdam Symptom Checklist (RSCL)

The 30 item checklist contains Likert type items that assess physical and psychosocial domains, and is completed by the patient.

Worthing Chemotherapy Questionnaire

The scale contains 75 Likert type items that assess physical, psychological, presence, severity, duration, and frequency domains associated with chemotherapy administration. The scale is completed by the patient.

Fig. 1. Comprehensive cancer symptom assessment instruments with acceptable psychometric properties. (*Data from* Kirkova J, Davis MP, Walsh D, et al. Cancer symptom assessment instruments: a systematic review. J Clin Oncol 2006;24:1459–73.)

identified by analyzing large symptom datasets and conducting either a factor or hierarchical cluster analysis of the data. Symptom domains, such as severity, frequency, or distress, can be included in the analysis. Statistically obtained clusters may suggest a common pathophysiology of the symptoms in the cluster [11].

Factors that impact symptoms and their relationship to one another include the stage of disease, treatment, treatment modifications (eg, dose or schedule adjustments), presence of comorbidities, and psychologic, sociologic, and cultural factors [14–16]. Research in the area of symptom clusters is relatively new and needed to develop reliable clinical assessment tools [17].

A study of 518 patients with bone metastases addressed the question of whether bone pain clustered with other symptoms. Pain was experienced by most patients and clustered with fatigue, drowsiness, and poor sense of well-being [18]. Similarly, in a study of 73 patients with gliomas, the four co-occurring symptoms of pain, fatigue, sleep disturbance, and depression significantly correlated with one another [19]. In another study, 51 patients with lung cancer had a symptom cluster that consisted of depression and fatigue [20].

Symptom clusters may have a common underlying cause. Determining causation aids in symptom management. In one study, symptoms clustered into three groups: pain eelated (pain, fatigue, sleep disturbance, lack of appetite, and drowsiness), chemotherapy related (nausea and vomiting), and emotion related (distress, sadness, depression). Identifying underlying causes of symptoms can help identify targeted nursing interventions. For instance, if insomnia causes fatigue and exacerbates pain, it may be possible that fatigue could be reduced by managing insomnia and pain [3].

The concept of symptom clusters, rather than symptoms occurring in isolation, better reflects the reality of the symptom experience, opens new areas of investigation, and may help explain contradictory findings of previous research. More research is needed to explore biologic and other mechanisms associated with symptom clusters, such as inflammatory pathways (specifically proinflammatory cytokine production). Improved symptom management may reduce polypharmacy, lessen drug side effects, and have pharmacoeconomic benefits. There are many study design and research issues, however, such as sample selection, timing of measures of symptoms, control of symptom interventions, which symptoms to evaluate, methods of scaling symptoms, and time frame of responses [21–23].

Symptom burden

"Symptom burden" is a term used to describe symptoms and their impact on patients' lives. A concept analysis of symptom burden identified multiple symptoms related to worsening disease as the major antecedent for the concept. Consequences of symptom burden include decreased survival, poor prognosis, treatment delay or discontinuation, increased hospitalizations and medical costs, decreased function, and lowered self-reported quality of life (QOL) [24]. Symptom burden goes beyond symptom assessment and includes the impact of symptoms on patients' lives, such as distress associated with the symptoms and interference with daily activities. Symptom burden can be used as an alternative to QOL measures or as a supplement to QOL measures [25].

Symptom burden and QOL measures provide meaningful but conceptually different data. QOL is a multidimensional construct that contains physical, emotional, and social domains. Symptoms contribute to, but do not determine, QOL. Conversely, QOL instruments are not intended to be symptom measurement instruments, although many QOL measures contain items related to patients' symptoms [9].

Research on symptom burden associated with specific types of cancer or cancer treatment is emerging. For instance, the symptom burden of patients with renal cell carcinoma depends on stage of disease, with patients who have localized disease reporting that irritability and pain occurred most often, whereas patients with metastatic disease experienced fatigue and weakness most often [26]. The symptom burden of patients undergoing stem cell transplantation includes lack of appetite, fatigue, weakness, sleep disturbance, nausea, and diarrhea. These symptoms affected all aspects of the patients' lives [27].

As increasing numbers of people live with cancer, clinicians and researchers are challenged to find assessment tools that can be used over time—in some cases, long periods of time (eg, with childhood cancer survivors). With respect to cancer survivorship, symptom burden assessment provides information about persistent symptoms, their severity, and their impact on patients' survivorship experiences. Symptom burden may be a better approach to studying late and long-term effects of cancer treatment, which have historically been understudied, than traditional single-symptom or QOL measures [28].

Symptom management across the disease continuum

Management of symptoms depends on the context in which the symptoms arise. For instance, the symptom of pain is assessed and managed differently in the immediate postoperative period than at the end of life. Anorexia that occurs on the day after chemotherapy is assessed and managed differently than anorexia that has been present for months in a patient who is newly diagnosed with pancreatic cancer. Much of the research on symptoms as they relate to a specific phase of the disease process has been conducted on symptoms that occur at the end of life. Patients who have cancer are confronted with increasing numbers of symptoms during the final months of their lives. Prevalent symptoms include fatigue, anorexia, malaise, anxiety, and loneliness. In clinical practice, physical symptoms are more often treated than psychosocial symptoms, so greater attention to patients' well-being is needed [29,30]. Families of patients who have cancer also report significant symptoms associated with caring for relatives at the end of life [31].

In one study, symptoms experienced by 922 patients with advanced cancer were categorized as fatigue (anorexia-cachexia), neuropsychological, upper gastrointestinal, nausea and vomiting, aerodigestive, debility, and pain. The researchers suggest that recognizing symptom clusters that occur at the end of life can help understand symptom pathophysiology and identify therapies that relieve multiple symptoms. This approach has the potential to reduce the number of medications that patients receive, potentially decrease medication-related side effects, and be more cost-effective than treating individual symptoms [4].

Although most children who have cancer are cured of their disease, some children experience disease progression or treatment complications and require palliative care. Managing symptoms during this time is challenging and is best accomplished using a family-centered approach [32].

Even cancer survivors have symptom management needs; common sequelae of cancer treatment include fatigue, cognitive changes, fear of recurrence, anxiety, stress syndromes, symptoms related to sexual and reproductive function, body image disturbance, and others. Psychosocial interventions, particularly group-based interventions and physical activity programs, have shown success in managing these symptoms for many patients [33]. In another study that examined symptoms in the context of employment, 328 cancer survivors reported symptoms of fatigue and stress that impacted their ability to work and relationships with their employers and co-workers [34].

The optimal schedule for assessing patients' symptoms is unknown and probably varies by clinical setting. Some symptom assessment instruments are appropriate for initial assessment but may be too lengthy or cumbersome for routine follow-up use or inappropriate for use at the end of life. Although repeated assessments provide a more accurate measurement of change over time, symptoms may change rapidly and unexpectedly. Some patients may become physically or emotionally distressed and unable to complete a symptom assessment instrument. Assisted assessment may be appropriate with distressed patients and patients whose clinical status prevents them from completing a self-assessment instrument. Some patients (eg, dying patients) also may be unable to participate in any type of symptom measurement [9].

Symptom management across the lifespan

Children

Children report symptoms as the most troublesome aspect of cancer treatment [35]. A review of published research studies found that the symptoms experienced most often by children with cancer were pain, nausea and vomiting, nutrition-related problems, mucositis, and fatigue [36]. These symptoms cause distress, are prevalent, are usually multiple, and may interfere with a child's growth and development [37]. Symptom distress is higher among inpatients, children with solid tumors, and children who are undergoing treatment as compared with children who have completed cancer treatment [38].

Most studies of children's symptom experiences have focused on individual symptoms, and, in many cases, measurement instruments were adapted from those designed for adults. In many cases, symptom terminology has been changed to be more age appropriate. For instance, "feeling nervous" is often used instead of the word "anxiety." Future studies need longitudinal designs that conceptualizes the symptom experience from the perspective of the child and measure clusters of symptoms at multiple levels (eg, emotional, behavioral, and biophysiologic). Attention also needs to be given to factors such as family dynamics, social networks, school and community influences, and the health care system, because each of them likely influences the symptom experience of children with cancer [39].

Older adults

Although people aged 65 years and older comprise the fastest growing segment of the United States population, little research on the symptom experience of older adults with cancer has been conducted. Few tools to measure symptoms have been developed and tested. Because older patients with cancer are in physiologic decline and typically have comorbidities, it is difficult to determine if symptoms are caused by cancer, other diseases, cancer treatment, treatment of other diseases, or a combination of any or all of these factors [40]. As noted earlier, stage of disease influences the symptom experience.

A study conducted at 24 sites found that later stages of cancer, multiple comorbid conditions, and being treated with chemotherapy were significant predictors of symptoms reported by 220 older patients with lung cancer (mean age, 72 years). There also was a correlation among the number of symptoms reported, the severity of the symptoms, and physical and functional limitations [41].

Older patients with advanced cancer often experience fatigue, pain, and depression. None of the tools to measure these symptoms have been tested in the older patient with advanced cancer. Treatment of fatigue in this age and disease group may involve education, antidepressants, treatment of anemia, exercise, and use of psychostimulants. Pain should be assessed systematically; the Visual Descriptor Scale, which contains a set of numbers with words representing different levels of pain, is the tool most preferred by older patients. Pain management in older patients may include acetaminophen, nonsteroidal anti-inflammatory drugs, opioids, adjuvant analgesics, and education of patients and caregivers. Depression is also a prevalent symptom that arises from various causes and often occurs simultaneously with fatigue and pain [42,43].

Comprehensive geriatric oncology assessments are designed to assess patients' symptoms and needs in the context of the patients' wishes about the aggressiveness or extensiveness of treatment. Research is needed on the occurrence, prevalence, and interdisciplinary management of symptoms that occur in older patients with cancer [44]. Research also may help determine how cancer, comorbidities, and the aging process interrelate and interact with one another to impact the patients' symptom experience.

Evidenced-based symptom management

The focus on evidence to guide nursing practice is gaining momentum in the United States and other countries. Evidence-based practice de-emphasizes ritual and tradition-based care and instead stresses the use of research findings as the basis for practice. The need for evidence-based practice was sparked by the Institute of Medicine's 1999 report, "To Err is Human" [45].

Although the highest level of evidence is well-designed randomized controlled trials conducted at multiple sites (Table 1), this level of evidence does not exist for many aspects of nursing practice, including symptom management of patients with cancer. It is critical to rely on the best available knowledge to inform patient care. Rutledge and Grant [46] explained that evidence-based practice, "defines care that integrates best scientific evidence with clinical expertise, knowledge of pathophysiology, knowledge of psychosocial issues, and decision making preferences of patients."

Within the arena of evidence-based practice, nurses must be ever conscious of the contribution of nursing care to patient outcomes, which are also called "nursing-sensitive patient outcomes." According to the Oncology Nursing Society, "nursing-sensitive patient outcomes are those outcomes arrived at, or significantly impacted by, nursing interventions. The interventions must be within the scope of nursing practice and integral to the processes of nursing care; an empiric link must exist" [47]. Nursing-sensitive patient outcomes are impacted by care that is rendered in collaboration with other health care providers. These outcomes represent the consequences or effects of nursing interventions and can result in changes in patient's symptom experience, functional status, safety, psychologic distress, and costs.

Table 1
Oncology Nursing Society levels of evidence

Oncology Nursing Society level	Source of evidence
I	Meta-analysis of multiple, well-designed, controlled studies, experimental studies, and well-designed, nonrandomized studies
II	Systematic reviews of nonexperimental studies
III	Non–research-based evidence derived from qualitative studies, case reports, and expert opinion

Legislators, regulators, insurers, and consumers want to be assured that patient care has "value" (cost effectively produces positive outcomes or improvement in health status). Because cancer treatment is associated with high costs, oncology nurses have tremendous opportunity to prevent or minimize symptoms associated with cancer and its treatment and, by doing so, help control health care costs.

Evidence-based resources

National Comprehensive Cancer Network

A variety of organizations and groups have recognized the need for evidence-based oncology practice. The National Comprehensive Network (NCCN), a not-for-profit alliance of 21 of the leading cancer centers in the United States, is dedicated to improving the quality and effectiveness of care provided to patients with cancer. The NCCN has developed and continuously updates clinical practice guidelines on cancer treatment; guidelines for the detection, prevention, and risk reduction of cancer; and guidelines for supportive care (Fig. 2).

NCCN Clinical Practice Guidelines in Oncology (available at www.nccn.org) are systematically developed statements that assist health care providers and patients make decisions about appropriate health care for specific clinical circumstances [48]. The development of the guidelines is based on evaluation of available scientific evidence with the expert judgment of leading clinicians from NCCN. Table 2 provides the categories of evidence outlined by NCCN and the strength of the evidence needed to meet the criteria for specific categories. In the NCCN guidelines for supportive care, most of the recommendations are category 2A, in which there is a lower level of evidence than category I, but there is a high level of consensus among the panel members based on the available evidence or practitioner experience. For example, in the clinical practice guideline on cancer-related fatigue, the recommendations for general strategies for the management of fatigue (eg, delegating, pacing activities, taking naps that do not interrupt nighttime sleep) are all examples of category 2A evidence. Based on these data, evidence exists to teach patients these energy-conserving activities for the management of fatigue.

Adult cancer pain
Antiemesis
Cancer- and cancer treatment-related anemia
Cancer related fatigue
Distress management
Myeloid growth factors
Palliative care
Pediatric cancer pain
Prevention and treatment of cancer-related infections
Senior adult oncology
Thromboembolic disease

Fig. 2. Available NCCN guidelines for supportive care.

Table 2
National Comprehensive Network categories of evidence and consensus

Category of evidence and consensus	Quality of evidence	Level of consensus
1. High-level evidence: high-powered randomized clinical trials or meta-analyses	High	Uniform
2A. Lower-level evidence: phase II or large cohort studies to individual practitioner experience; some recommendations are based on consensus of experience-based opinion	Lower	Uniform
2B. Lower-level evidence: evidence from studies is not conclusive, thus more than one approach can be inferred from the existing data	Lower	Nonuniform
3. Level of evidence is not pertinent in this category. Major interpretation issue related to the data, thus no specific recommendation made overall	Any	Major disagreement

National Comprehensive Network, 2007.

Oncology Nursing Society

The Oncology Nursing Society values and supports evidence-based practice to guide clinical management of patients with cancer. It has developed a set of evidence-based resources for use by staff nurses, advanced practice nurses, and nurse researchers. These resources, called the "Putting Evidence into Practice" (PEP) resources, focus (to date) on symptom management of the patient and their family with cancer (Fig. 3). Available resources include PEP quick reference cards, detailed PEP reference cards, definitions of the terms used to define the evidence, evidence tables that support the levels of evidence assigned to each of the interventions, tables of guidelines that were used in the assignment of the level of evidence to interventions, meta-analyses tables of the evidence, references used in the development of the resources, and summaries of measurement of the outcomes specific to oncology patients (including table of instruments recommended for

Fatigue
Dyspnea
Mucositis
Depression
Constipation
Peripheral Neuropathy
Prevention of Infection
Sleep-Wake Disturbances
Caregiver Strain and Burden
Chemotherapy-Induced Nausea and Vomiting

Fig. 3. Available PEP resources.

measurement of the outcome). All of these resources are available at www.ons.org/outcomes.

The categories of evidence for each of the interventions reviewed in the PEP resources are based on the Oncology Nursing Society levels of evidence (Table 3) but have been further defined for the purposes of the resources. For the purposes of the PEP quick reference cards, the interventions are presented according to color coding. The idea of this color coding is that it allows the clinician to quickly identify the strength of the evidence for particular interventions. Interventions placed in the green categories are interventions for which high level evidence exists, thus they are "recommended for practice" or "likely to be effective." Interventions placed in the yellow categories are interventions for which lower levels of evidence exist, or the evidence for an intervention may not yet be established. These interventions are categorized as "benefits balanced with harms" or "effectiveness not established." Interventions that are categorized in the red category have even lesser levels of evidence to support their recommendation or are interventions for which clear evidence has demonstrated ineffectiveness or harmfulness. These interventions are categorized as "effectiveness unlikely" or "not recommended for practice."

An example of how the PEP resources can be used in clinical practice is when a patient is experiencing fatigue. The nurse could refer to the quick reference card titled, "What interventions are effective in preventing and

Table 3
Oncology Nursing Society categories of evidence for the "putting evidence into practice" resources

Category of evidence	Support for category of evidence
Green: recommended for practice	High level evidence: rigorously designed studies, meta-analyses, or systematic reviews
Green: likely to be effective	High level evidence, but evidence is less well established than for "recommended for practice"
Yellow: benefits balanced with harms	Lower level of evidence than for the green categories; the benefits and harmful effects of the interventions should be weighed according to individual circumstance
Yellow: effectiveness not established	Lower level of evidence than for the green categories; interventions in which insufficient evidence or inadequate quality of data exists
Red: effectiveness unlikely	Low level of evidence; there is a lack of effectiveness less well established than for the interventions listed in "not recommended for practice"
Red: not recommended for practice	High level of evidence demonstrated for the ineffectiveness or harmfulness of interventions or where the cost or burden for the intervention exceeds the benefit

treating fatigue during and following cancer and its treatment" [49]. Under "recommended for practice" the nurse would find that exercise has been found (according to high level evidence) to help prevent and manage fatigue during and after cancer treatment in patients with breast cancer and solid tumors and patients undergoing hematopoietic stem cell transplantation. The nurse could also find more information about the types of exercise that were studied in these patient populations on the quick reference card. Using the Internet-based data regarding the PEP resources, the nurse could find the references to support the intervention and supporting data for all of the interventions on the quick reference card.

Multinational Association of Supportive Care in Cancer and the International Society of Oral Oncology

The Multinational Association of Supportive Care in Cancer (MASCC) was founded in 1991 and formally joined the International Society of Oral Oncology (ISOO) in 1998. The purpose of MASCC is to "optimize supportive care in cancer patients worldwide, stimulate multi-disciplinary research, encourage international scientific exchange of information, expand professional expertise in supportive care, educate health care professionals worldwide in supportive care, and to serve as a resource for patients, families, and caregivers" [50]. MASCC/ISOO has several Internet-based resource centers on topics such as fatigue, infection, mucositis, and skin toxicities. These resource centers house information from working group meetings, information about conferences and symposiums devoted to the symptom, and related publications. The symptoms that have been developed and have published evidence-based guidelines include antiemetic therapy, myelosuppression, and mucositis (www.mascc.org). The MASCC categories of evidence include the MASCC level of confidence and the MASCC level of consensus. An example of the categories of evidence is related to the guidelines for the prevention of acute nausea and vomiting after chemotherapy of high emetogenic risk. MASCC guidelines recommend using a three-drug combination regimen that includes a 5-HT3 antagonist, dexamethasone, and aprepitant given before the chemotherapy. The MASCC level of confidence for this recommendation is high and the level of consensus is high.

Use of evidence-based guidelines

Although much effort has gone into the development of evidence-based clinical practice guidelines, little is actually known about their use and effectiveness. Most of the efforts of the NCCN are in the development of the cancer treatment guidelines and not in the evaluation of use. The PEP resources developed by the Oncology Nursing Society are relatively new, and no evaluative efforts have been made to date regarding their use or effectiveness. The Oncology Nursing Society is reviewing methods by which to evaluate the PEP resources. McGuire and colleagues [51] published survey results of health care professional's awareness of the MASCC/ISOO mucositis management guidelines that were published in 2004. They surveyed a select group of health care professionals (attendees at three cancer-related professional conferences) and found a significant lack of awareness of the guidelines: only approximately one third of the US respondents were aware of the 2004 guidelines compared with approximately 80% of the European respondents. It is clear that organizations and individual practitioners need to develop strategies to disseminate the clinical practice guidelines, enhance awareness and use of guidelines, and develop patient teaching tools based on these evidence-based guidelines.

Complementary and alternative symptom management

Complementary therapies are therapies used in conjunction with conventional treatment. Alternative therapies are used in place of conventional treatment and are usually implemented by patients when conventional treatment does not bring satisfactory relief or causes undesirable side effects. Integrated or integrative care is a growing field in which patients and health care providers work together to develop a plan of care that draws on a variety of traditions, expertise, and modalities to address an individual's specific needs. Care plans developed in this framework may include one or more treatment modalities, pharmacologic and nonpharmacologic therapies, and referrals to other practitioners [52].

Complementary, alternative, and integrative therapies often are used by patients to manage symptoms associated with cancer and its treatment. These therapies are used by 31% to 84% of children with cancer, including many children enrolled in clinical trials [53], and are estimated to be used by 55% of adults with cancer [54]. Patients do not always report use of these therapies, however [55].

Although many of the complementary, alternative, and integrative therapies are helpful adjunctive approaches that help control symptoms and enhance QOL, some therapies are inefficacious or harmful. Health care providers need to be aware of popularly used therapies and know where to find reliable information for themselves and their patients [56]. One resource is the National Cancer Institute (NCI) Office of Cancer Complementary and Alternative Medicine (CAM) (www.nci.nih.gov/cam), which was established to coordinate and enhance activities of the NCI in CAM research as it relates to the prevention, diagnosis, and treatment of cancer, cancer-related symptoms, and side effects of conventional cancer treatment.

CAM research in symptom management largely consists of small, nonrandomized studies. Increasing numbers of randomized controlled studies are being conducted, however. Controlled clinical trials found that acupuncture and hypnotherapy can reduce the cancer-related symptoms of pain and nausea. Meditation, relaxation therapy, music therapy, and massage are helpful in reducing anxiety and distress. Herbs, botanicals, and dietary supplements are commonly used therapies but may be problematic, so the risks and benefits of using these products in conjunction with conventional treatment, such as chemotherapy, must be investigated and considered [57].

A review of research studies examining the use of CAM among children with cancer found that small clinical study findings suggested that acupuncture and ginger are effective in treating nausea and vomiting, and hypnosis and imagery are effective for treating pain and anxiety. Larger randomized trials are needed to further explore the role of CAM in pediatric symptom management [58].

Until more evidence is available, health care providers need to specifically ask about and document CAM use. Patients may not realize that a "natural" remedy for nausea, such as herbal tea that contains large amounts of ginger and red clover, may have adverse effects on blood clotting. Health care providers also need to evaluate the evidence or lack of evidence for CAM therapies, discuss the potential benefits and risks of CAM use with patients, and assist patients in making informed decisions about CAM use.

Summary

Symptoms experienced by patients with cancer may be disease-related, treatment-related, related to comorbid conditions, or a combination of all three. Patients typically experience symptoms in multiples, and often these symptoms are interrelated or cluster. Multidimensional measurement scales that incorporate the most common symptoms are needed to help ensure systematic assessment. Optimally, valid and reliable tools that measure symptom clusters could be used in clinical and research settings. Studying the complex symptoms associated with cancer and its treatment may yield increased understanding of patterns of association, interaction, and synergy of symptoms and result in improved clinical outcomes [2,13].

References

[1] Dodd MJ, Cho MH, Cooper B, et al. Advancing our knowledge of symptom clusters. J Support Oncol 2005;3(6 Suppl 4):30–1.

[2] Barsevick AM. The elusive concept of the symptom cluster. Oncol Nurs Forum 2007;34:971–80.

[3] Chen ML, Tseng HH. Identification and verification of symptom clusters in cancer patients. J Support Oncol 2005;3(6 Suppl 4):28–9.

[4] Walsh D, Rybicki L. Symptom clustering in advanced cancer. Support Care Cancer 2006;14:831–6.

[5] Wedding U, Roehrig B, Klippstein A, et al. Comorbidity in patients with cancer: prevalence and severity measured by cumulative illness rating scale. Crit Rev Oncol Hematol 2007;61:269–76.

[6] Lorenz KA, Lynn J, Dy S, et al. Quality measures for symptoms and advance care planning in cancer: a systematic review. J Clin Oncol 2006;24:4933–8.

[7] Surbone A, Kagawa-Singer M, Terret C, et al. The illness trajectory of elderly cancer patients across cultures: SIOG position paper. Ann Oncol 2007;18:633–8.
[8] Patrick DL, Ferketich SL, Frame PS, et al. National Institutes of Health State-of-the-Science Conference Statement. Symptom management in cancer: pain, depression, and fatigue. July 15-17, 2002. J Natl Cancer Inst Monogr 2004;(32):9–16.
[9] Kirkova J, Davis MP, Walsh D, et al. Cancer symptom assessment instruments: a systematic review. J Clin Oncol 2006;24:1459–73.
[10] Barsevick AM. The concept of symptom cluster. Semin Oncol Nurs 2007;23:89–98.
[11] Kirkova J, Walsh D. Cancer symptom clusters: a dynamic construct. Support Care Cancer 2007;15:1011–3.
[12] Kim HJ, McGuire DB, Tulman L, et al. Symptom clusters: concept analysis and clinical implications for nursing. Cancer Nurs 2005;28:270–82.
[13] Barsevick AM, Whitmer K, Nail LM, et al. Symptom cluster research: conceptual, design, measurement, and analysis issues. J Pain Symptom Manage 2006;31:85–95.
[14] Gift AG. Symptom clusters related to specific cancers. Semin Oncol Nurs 2007;23:136–41.
[15] Honea N, Brant J, Beck SL. Treatment-related symptom clusters. Semin Oncol Nurs 2007; 23:142–51.
[16] Given BA, Given CW, Sikorskii A, et al. Symptom clusters and physical function for patients receiving chemotherapy. Semin Oncol Nurs 2007;23:121–6.
[17] Lacasse C, Beck SL. Clinical assessment of symptom clusters. Semin Oncol Nurs 2007;23: 106–12.
[18] Chow E, Fan G, Hadi S, et al. Symptom clusters in cancer patients with bone metastases. Support Care Cancer 2007;15:1035–43.
[19] Fox SW, Lyon D, Farace E. Symptom clusters in patients with high-grade glioma. J Nurs Scholarsh 2007;39:61–7.
[20] Fox SW, Lyon DE. Symptom clusters and quality of life in survivors of lung cancer. Oncol Nurs Forum 2006;33:931–6.
[21] Chen ML, Lin CC. Cancer symptom clusters: a validation study. J Pain Symptom Manage 2007;34:590–9.
[22] Miaskowski C, Aouizerat BE. Is there a biological basis for the clustering of symptoms? Semin Oncol Nurs 2007;23:99–105.
[23] Williams LA. Clinical management of symptom clusters. Semin Oncol Nurs 2007;23:113–20.
[24] Gapstur RL. Symptom burden: a concept analysis and implications for oncology nurses. Oncol Nurs Forum 2007;34:673–80.
[25] Cleeland CS, Reyes-Gibby CC. When is it justified to treat symptoms? Measuring symptom burden. Oncology 2002;16(9 Suppl 10):64–70.
[26] Harding G, Cella D, Robinson D, et al. Symptom burden among patients with renal cell carcinoma (RCC): content for a symptom index. Health Qual Life Outcomes 2007;5:34.
[27] Anderson KO, Giralt SA, Mendoza TR, et al. Symptom burden in patients undergoing autologous stem-cell transplantation. Bone Marrow Transplant 2007;39:759–66.
[28] Burkett VS, Cleeland CS. Symptom burden in cancer survivorship. Journal of Cancer Survivorship 2007;1:167–75.
[29] Georges JJ, Onwuteaka-Philipsen BD, van der Heide A, et al. Symptoms, treatment and "dying peacefully" in terminally ill cancer patients: a prospective study. Support Care Cancer 2005;13:160–8.
[30] Jocham HR, Dassen T, Widdershoven G, et al. Quality of life in palliative care cancer patients: a literature review. J Clin Nurs 2006;15:1188–95.
[31] Lagman R, Walsh D. Integration of palliative medicine into comprehensive care. Semin Oncol 2005;32:134–8.
[32] Friedman DL, Hilden JM, Powaski K. Issues and challenges in palliative care for children with cancer. Curr Pain Headache Rep 2005;9:249–55.
[33] Alfano CM, Rowland JH. Recovery issues in cancer survivorship: a new challenge for supportive care. Cancer J 2006;12:432–43.

[34] Pryce J, Munir F, Haslam C. Cancer survivorship and work: symptoms, supervisor response, co-worker disclosure and work adjustment. J Occup Rehabil 2007;17:83–92.
[35] Rheingans JI. A systematic review of nonpharmacologic adjunctive therapies for symptom management in children with cancer. J Pediatr Oncol Nurs 2007;24:81–94.
[36] Hockenberry M. Symptom management research in children with cancer. J Pediatr Oncol Nurs 2004;21:132–6.
[37] Hockenberry M, Hooke MC. Symptom clusters in children with cancer. Semin Oncol Nurs 2007;23:152–7.
[38] Collins JJ, Byrnes ME, Dunkel IJ, et al. The measurement of symptoms in children with cancer. J Pain Symptom Manage 2000;19:363–77.
[39] Docherty SL. Symptom experiences of children and adolescents with cancer. Annu Rev Nurs Res 2003;21:123–49.
[40] Satariano WA, Silliman RA. Comorbidity: implications for research and practice in geriatric oncology. Crit Rev Oncol Hematol 2003;48:239–48.
[41] Gift AG, Jablonski A, Stommel M, et al. Symptom clusters in elderly patients with lung cancer. Oncol Nurs Forum 2004;31:202–12.
[42] Rao A, Cohen HJ. Symptom management in the elderly cancer patient: fatigue, pain, and depression. J Natl Cancer Inst Monographs 2004;32:150–7.
[43] White H. The older cancer patient. Med Clin North Am 2003;90:967–82.
[44] Terret C, Zulian GB, Naiem A, et al. Multidisciplinary approach to the geriatric oncology patient. J Clin Oncol 2007;10:1876–81.
[45] Kohn LT, Corrigan JM, Donalson MS, Institute of Medicine. To err is human: building a safer health system. Washington, DC: National Academy Press; 2000.
[46] Rutledge DN, Grant M. Evidence-based practice in cancer nursing: introduction. Semin Oncol Nurs 2002;18:1–2.
[47] Given B, Beck S, Etland C, et al. Nursing-sensitive patient outcomes. Available at: http://www.ons.org/outcomes/measures/outcomes.html. Accessed September 8, 2007.
[48] Field MJ, Lohr KN, editors. Clinical practice guidelines: direction for a new program. Institute of Medicine, Committee on Clinical Practice Guidelines. Washington, DC: National Academy Press; 1990.
[49] Mitchell S, Beck S, Hood L, et al. What interventions are effective in preventing and treating fatigue during and following cancer and its treatment? Oncology Nursing Society; PEP Quick Reference Card, 2005.
[50] Herrstedt J. New aspects of supportive care: the MASCC vision. Arch Oncol 2004;12:161–2.
[51] McGuire DB, Johnson J, Migliorati C. Promulgation of guidelines for mucositis management: educating healthcare professionals and patients. Support Care Cancer 2006; 14:548–51.
[52] Hess DJ. Complementary or alternative? Stronger vs weaker integration policies. Am J Public Health 2002;92:1579–81.
[53] Kelly KM. Complementary and alternative medical therapies for children with cancer. Eur J Cancer 2004;40:2041–6.
[54] Saydah SH, Eberhardt MS. Use of complementary and alternative medicine among adults with chronic diseases: United States 2002. J Altern Complement Med 2006;12: 805–12.
[55] Given SM, Liberman N, Klang S, et al. Are people who use "natural drugs" aware of their potentially harmful side effects and reporting to family physicians? Patient Educ Couns 2004; 53:5–11.
[56] Cassileth BR, Deng G. Complementary and alternative therapies for cancer. Oncologist 2004;9:80–9.
[57] Deng G, Cassileth BR, Yeung KS. Complementary therapies for cancer-related symptoms. J Support Oncol 2004;2:419–26.
[58] Ladas EJ, Post-White J, Hawks R, et al. Evidence for symptom management in the child with cancer. J Pediatr Hematol Oncol 2006;28:601–15.

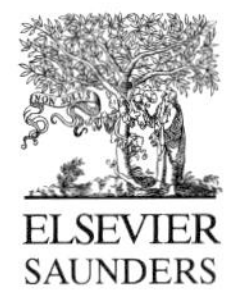

ELSEVIER
SAUNDERS

Nurs Clin N Am 43 (2008) 221–241

NURSING
CLINICS
OF NORTH AMERICA

The Marriage of Conventional Cancer Treatments and Alternative Cancer Therapies

Georgia M. Decker, MS, APRN-BC, CN, AOCN

Integrative Care, N.P., P.C., Albany, NY, USA

The history of complementary and alternative therapies precedes the nineteenth century, when unconventional methods of disease treatment with the intent to cure were considered and termed "folk medicine" or "quackery." Practitioners of this first generation of alternative medicine systems in the early twentieth century (eg, Thomsonianism, homeopathy, mesmerism, eclectism) shared theoretic principles and therapeutic strategies [1]. Establishing societies, journals, and schools provided increased credibility to these systems, which allowed for the recruitment of approximately 10% of the practice field. Hahnemann, founder of the system of homeopathy that became popular in the United States in the 1830s, coined the term "allopathic," which is currently a standard term for orthodox or conventional medicine. A second generation of developing systems (eg, osteopathy, chiropractic, naturopathy) was established by the late twentieth, century realizing an estimated 20% of all medical practice. Contemporary holism appeared simultaneously and focused on treating the "whole" patient [1]. Therapeutic interventions relying on natural healing (nineteenth century term), drugless healing (early twentieth century term), or holistic healing (1970s to the present term) were not unique to the United States.

The terms "alternative" or "unconventional" have been used to describe any therapy used instead of conventional approaches. Conventional approaches, known as "standard" or "traditional" or "biomedical" approaches, have had broad application in Western medicine. Complementary and alternative medicine (CAM) has been referred to as "integrative," "integrated," or "complementary" when therapies are combined with conventional approaches. A therapy is not "alternative" or "complementary" by definition. It is the intended use that describes and defines a therapy [2–4].

E-mail address: jorja@att.net

doi:10.1016/j.cnur.2008.02.006

That is, a particular therapy may be considered complementary (to complement a conventional therapy) or alternative (instead of conventional therapy). The interchangeable use of the terms alternative and complementary has contributed to misunderstanding and miscommunication [3–5]. The terms "integrated" or "integrative" are the most contemporary.

National surveys demonstrate a sustained interest in and use of these therapies [6–8]. In an effort to address the use of these therapies and issues surrounding their use, the Office of Alternative Medicine was established at the National Institutes of Health (NIH) by the United States Congress in 1992 and later became the National Center for Complementary and Alternative Medicine (NCCAM) in 1998. NCCAM is one of the 27 institutes and centers that make up the NIH. NCCAM has four primary focus areas: research (clinical and basic science research), training and career development (pre-doctoral, postdoctoral, and career researchers), outreach (conferences, educational programs, and exhibits, information clearinghouse), and integration (scientifically proven CAM practices into conventional medicine) [9,10]. The National Cancer Institute (NCI) established the Office of Cancer Complementary and Alternative Medicine (OCCAM) within the Office of the Director in 1998 in an effort to increase high quality research and information associated with the use of CAM. The OCCAM promotes and supports research within CAM disciplines and therapies as they relate to the prevention, diagnosis, and treatment of cancer, cancer-related symptoms, and side effects of conventional treatment. The OCCAM coordinates research, informational activities, and collaboration with other governmental and nongovernmental organizations on cancer CAM issues by the NCI. OCCAM also provides an interface with health care practitioners and researchers regarding cancer CAM issues [5,11,12].

The White House Commission on Complementary and Alternative Medicine Policy was established in March 2000 to address issues related to access and delivery of CAM, priorities for research, and the need for consumer and health care provider (HCP) education. The Commission endorsed ten principles (Box 1) [13]. The Institute of Medicine of the National Academies, a nongovernmental agency, guarantees unbiased, evidence-based information and advice concerning health and science policy to policymakers, HCP, and the public. In 2003 to 2004, the Institute of Medicine committee met to explore scientific, policy, and practice questions that arise from the increasing use of CAM by the American public [14].

Use of complementary and alternative medicine in the United States

Understanding the use of CAM in the United States includes various related issues, including the reasons for using CAM (motive), the frequency with which use occurs (prevalence), and the people who use it (patient characteristics) [15,16]. Other authors report additional reasons for the revitalization of complementary and alternative medicine in the twenty-first

Box 1. Guiding principles from the White House Commission on complementary and alternative medicine

A wholeness orientation in health care delivery: delivery of high-quality health care must support care of the whole person
Evidence of safety and efficacy: use science to generate evidence that protects and promotes public health
Healing capacity of a person: support capacity for recovery and self-healing
Respect for individuality: each person has the right to health care that is responsive, respects preferences, and preserves dignity
Right to choose treatment: each person has the right to choose freely among safe and effective approaches and among qualified practitioners
Emphasis on health promotion and self-care: good health care emphasizes self-care and early interventions for maintaining and promoting health
Partnerships in integrated health care: good health care requires teamwork among patients, HCP, and researchers committed to creating healing environments and respecting diversity of health care traditions
Education as a fundamental health care service: education about prevention, healthy lifestyles, and self-healing should be part of the curricular of all HCP and made available to the public
Dissemination of comprehensive, timely information: health care quality is enhanced by examination of the evidence on which CAM systems, practices, and products are based. This information should be widely, rapidly, and easily available
Integral public involvement: input from informed consumers must be incorporated in proposing priorities for health care, research, policy decisions

From White House Commission on Complementary and Alternative Medicine. Available at: www.whccamp.hhs.gov. Accessed September 17, 2007.

century in the United States, including philosophical similarity (emphasis on holism, active patient role, natural treatments, spiritual dimension), personal control over treatment, positive relationship with therapist (time for discussion, including emotional aspects), accessible, and increased well-being [9]. Possible factors contributing to the decreased use of conventional medicine in favor of CAM are dissatisfaction with health care providers and current therapies, including poor communication and inadequate time with HCP, adverse effects of current treatment regimens), rejection by current

HCP, desperation, and cost of care [9]. Other authors suggest that the persuasive appeal of CAM is related to a perceived association of CAM with nature, focus on energy forces that promote vitalism, and likely union of the physical (medical) and spiritual (truth, values, morals) realms [8,15,16]. The twenty-first century has seen an emergence of a new kind of patient: those who express their desire to take control of their own health, actively participate in decisions related to health and wellness, and may choose treatment plans involving solely conventional biomedical, solely CAM, or a combination of both [15–17].

Early national surveys that highlighted the prevalence, cost of use, and pattern of CAM use were published in 1993, at which time one in three respondents used at least one "unconventional" therapy within the past year, and one third of these respondents sought providers for "unconventional" therapy [16–19]. In the early to mid 1990s, CAM surveys were not disease specific. Trends over the past decade show a gradual increased prevalence of CAM use among patients in the United States [9,18–21]. Toward the end of the 1990s, more was known about CAM use among cancer patients, rural populations, and elderly patients, and similar trends in use were seen [20–28]. Studies conducted since 2000 (sample size $N \geq 100$) measured CAM use in adults with cancer between 25% and 80% [21,24,25,29–32]. Compared with non-CAM users, individuals who use CAM are more likely to be female, better educated, and have higher incomes [17–20,33]. Using a cross-sectional design in women with gynecologic cancer, one study reported that characteristics associated with CAM use include annual incomes more than $30,000, cancer site of origin other than cervix, and use of CAM before cancer diagnosis [32]. Respondents reported their reasons for using CAM as (1) hope of improved well-being and (2) possible anti-cancer effects of the particular CAM modalities used.

Another recent study in which 82% of the participants reported using CAM at some time in their lives cited their reasons for CAM use as therapeutic interventions for medical conditions such as depression, anxiety, and insomnia [24]. Researchers concluded that the oncology community must improve patient-provider communication and initiate research to determine possible drug-herb-vitamin interactions [31]. Research has demonstrated that oncology nurses contribute a vital function in educating patients on the safe use of therapies and incorporating CAM modalities such as relaxation, imagery, or healing touch into cancer care [24,33].

Consumers of CAM therapies are interested in choosing their providers, integrating CAM therapies into conventional care, limiting out-of-pocket expenses, and expanding insurance coverage. What patients are willing to pay for CAM may indicate the value they place on these therapies [34,35]. Reported mean out-of-pocket payments per visit for certain therapies were $23.00 for herbal therapies, $33.00 for massage, $44.00 for acupuncture, and $49.00 for nutritional advice [34]. Nearly $27 billion (out-of-pocket) were estimated as spent on alternative medicine professional services between 1990 and 1997, reflecting an increase of 45.2%. Given the financial investment in CAM therapies, a question that endures for researchers is whether CAM therapies can provide the beneficial health outcomes to justify the expense [18,19,34,35].

Categorizing complementary and alternative medicine

There are two main approaches to categorizing CAM therapies. NCCAM classifies CAM therapies into five domains: (1) alternative medical systems, (2) mind-body interventions, (3) biologically based therapies, (4) manipulative and body-based methods, and (5) energy therapies. The NCI OCCAM expanded the NCCAM domains with additional categories for clarification: movement therapy, pharmacologic and biologic treatments with a subcategory of complex natural products.

Alternative medical systems are built on complete systems of theory and practice. Mind-body medicine uses various techniques designed to enhance the mind's capacity to affect bodily function and symptoms. Biologically based therapies in CAM use substances found in nature, such as herbs, foods, and vitamins. Manipulative and body-based methods in CAM are based on manipulation and movement of one or more parts of the body. Energy therapies involve the use of energy field and are of two types: biofield therapies and bioelectromagnetic-based therapies. Movement therapies are modalities used to improve patterns of bodily movement. Pharmacologic and biological therapies are drugs, vaccines, off-label use of prescription drugs, and other biologic interventions not yet accepted in mainstream medicine. Complex natural products, a subcategory of the prior category, consist of crude natural substances and unfractionated extracts from marine organisms used for healing and treatment of disease. NCI OCCAM classifications provide a functional structure for the enhanced understanding of CAM as a whole and cancer CAM as a subcomponent. Table 1 describes each domain as defined by the OCCAM and provides examples.

Evidence-based practice

The classification system developed by the NCI PDQ Adult Treatment Editorial Board ranks human cancer treatment studies according to the statistical strength of the study design and specific scientific strength of the treatment outcomes. This classification has been adapted for use in human studies involving CAM treatments. The strength of the evidence is rank ordered in descending order from one to four. Case series are the weakest form of study design. For some CAM modalities, case series may be the only available or practical information known because many are already in use and there is an absence of preclinical and clinical data. Most of CAM has not undergone clinical trials [10].

Table 1
National Cancer Institute Office of Cancer Complementary and Alternative Medicine domains of complementary and alternative medicine

Domain	Definition	Example(s)
Alternative medical Systems	Systems built on completed systems of theory and practice	Traditional Chinese medicine (acupuncture), Ayurveda, homeopathy, naturopathy
Manipulative and body-based methods	Methods based on manipulation and/or movement of the one or more parts of the body	Chiropractic, therapeutic massage, osteopathy, reflexology
Energy therapies	Therapies involving the use of energy fields	Reiki, therapeutic touch, healing touch magnet therapy
Mind-body interventions	Techniques designed to enhance the mind's capacity to affect bodily function and symptoms	Meditation, hypnosis, art therapy, biofeedback, imagery, relaxation therapy, support groups, music therapy, cognitive-behavioral therapy, prayer, dance therapy, psychoneuro-immunology, aromatherapy, pet therapy
Movement therapy	Modalities used to improve patterns of bodily movement	T'ai Chi, Feldenkrais, Hathayoga, Alexander Technique, dance therapy, QiGong, Rolfing, Trager Method
Nutritional therapeutics	The use of specific foods, supplements, or diets as cancer prevention or treatment strategies	Dietary regimens such as macrobiotics, Gerson therapy, Kelley/Gonzalez regimen, vitamins, macronutrients, supplements, antioxidants
Pharmacologic and biologic treatments	Drugs, complex natural products, vaccines, and other biologic interventions not Food and Drug Administration approved, off-label use of prescription drugs	Antineoplastons, 714-X, low-dose naltrexone, immunoaugmentative therapy, laetrile, hydrazine sulfate, New Castle Virus, melatonin, ozone therapy, thymus therapy, enzyme therapy
Complex natural products	Subcategory of pharmacologic and biologic treatments consisting of an assortment of plant samples (botanicals), extracts of crude natural substances, and un-fractionate extracts from marine organisms used for healing and treatment of disease	Herbs and herbal extracts, mixtures of tea polyphenols, shark cartilage, Essiac tea, cordyceps, Sun Soup, MGN-3

From Decker G, Lee C. Complementary and alternative medicine (CAM) therapies. In: Yarbro C, Frogge M, Goodman M, editors. Cancer nursing principles and practice. 6th edition. Sudbury (MA): Jones and Bartlett; 2005. p. 590–620; with permission.

Levels of evidence in CAM are generated in the same fashion as that of conventional medicine, beginning with clinical trials involving CAM modalities for the treatment of cancer and cancer-related side effects. The positive or negative clinical trial results form the foundation for systematic reviews and meta-analyses, which, in turn, impact the development of evidence-based practice, research use, and practice guidelines [5,12]. Levels of evidence are frequently used by organizations such as the NCI (clinical trials) and the ONS (PRISM project) and databases such as Natural Medicine Comprehensive Database (NMCD), Natural Standard Database (Natural Standard), and the Oxford Center for Evidence-based Medicine [36–39]. Table 2 compares the strength of study design, endpoints measured, and level of evidence scores for these databases.

In CAM research, the goal and major challenge are the same—to ensure a methodologically meticulous trial without compromising the modality in a manner that is incomplete or inappropriate. The continued challenge is not that randomized controlled trials (RCTs) be used but rather how best to apply RCT results [40]. EBP in CAM requires a delicate and complex balance [38,39]. The balanced view is that both conventional medicine and CAM have benefits and limitations and that all therapeutic interventions can be held to the same rigorous standards of evidenced-based medicine. Not all CAM can be easily measured through clinical research. Long [42] offered three measurement areas for inclusion to establish and maintain consistency and accuracy: (1) philosophy and practice in healing in the CAM modality, (2) relationship between the user and the practitioner, and (3) techniques used to enhance the healing process [41,42].

Commonly used complementary and alternative medicine therapies and levels of evidence

Acupuncture

Acupuncture has been and is currently used by many Americans and is performed by many physicians, dentists, and acupuncturists for various health conditions. Acupuncture is used most often in the treatment of pain. Typically acupuncture involves insertion of a thin needle into the skin in specific sites (acupoints) for therapeutic purposes. Acupoint stimulation may also occur via electrical current, laser, moxibustion, pressure, ultrasound, and vibration and is of Japanese, Korean, or Chinese type. The principle is that *qi* (pronounced “chee” and translated as meaning *energy*) is present at birth and maintained throughout life. *Qi* circulates throughout the body, and 12 meridians provide a major path for the flow of *qi*. There are approximately 350 acupoints along the 12 meridians, with additional acupoints that lie outside the meridian pathways. Health is a balance of yin and yang (opposite forces present in everyone). Disease or any medical condition is a result of imbalance, commonly as a result of a blockage or

Table 2
Common levels of evidence in cancer complementary and alternative medicine

	Strength of study design	Strength of endpoints measured	Level of evidence score
Center for Evidence-based Medicine Database (CEBM, 2004)	1a: SR of RCTs 1b: Individual RCT with narrow confidence interval 1c: All or none 2a: SR of cohort studies 2b: Individual cohort study (including low quality RCT) 2c: Outcomes research, ecologic studies 3a: SR of case-controlled studies 3b: Individual case-control study 4: Case-series & poor quality cohort & case-control studies 5: Expert opinion without explicit critical appraisal or based on physiology, bench research, or "first principles"	A: Consistent level 1 studies B: Consistent level 2 or 3 studies or extrapolation from level 1 studies C: Level 4 or extrapolation from level 2 or 3 studies D: Level 5 evidence of troublingly inconsistent or inconclusive studies of any level	1 A, B, C 2 A, B, C 3 A, B 4 5
Physician Data Query (NCI, 2004)	1 RCT (DB/NB) 2 Non-RCT 3 Case series 4 Best case series	A: Total Mortality B: CS-mortality C: QOL D: Indirect surrogates	1-4 joined with A-D Joining score for study design with strength of endpoints measured

Natural Standards Database (NaturalStandard, 2004)	A Strong scientific evidence B Good scientific evidence C Unclear or conflicting scientific evidence D Fair negative Scientific evidence F Strong negative scientific evidence Lack of evidence unable to evaluate efficacy due to lack of adequate human data	Quality of Study 0–2 Poor 3–4 Good 5 Excellent	A B C D F Lack of evidence
Natural Medicines Comprehensive Database (NMCD, 2004)	*Weight of evidence* ○ Low ○○ Moderate ○○ ○ High *Direction of evidence* ⇑ Clearly positive ⇗ Tentatively positive ⇒ Uncertain ⇘ Tentatively Negative ⇓ Clearly Negative *Serious safety concerns* YES: Serious events have been reported or are considered possible NO: Reports of serious events were not located and are considered unlikely		Weight of evidence Direction of evidence Serious safety concerns
Priority Symptom PRISM Project (Ropka & Spencer-Cisek, 2001)	1: SR or MA of multiple RCTs 2: $>$ 1 RCT N $>$100 3: $>$ 1 non-RCT 4: Qualitative SR nonexperimental 5: Case controlled 6: Correlational study or case series 7: NIH Consensus reports, practice guidelines 8: Qualitative designs, expert opinion		I: Level of evidence 1–3 II: Level of evidence 4–7 III: Level of evidence 8

deficiency of energy. The belief that stimulating the appropriate acupoints aids the body in correcting any imbalance in the flow of energy and restoring balance provides the foundation of acupuncture. The balance of energy and flow of *qi* may be identified before disease has developed; therefore, acupuncture has a role in the prevention of illness and maintenance of health. Acupuncture been integrated with allopathic and osteopathic medicine in the United States [43]. Acupuncture has been and continues to be used for pain and other disorders of the musculoskeletal system, headaches, stress, ENT conditions (including sinusitis, tinnitus, and vertigo), allergies, dental pain, addictions, and immune system support, among others [43–49].

Highlights of evidence

More than 30 meta-analysis (MA) or systematic review (SR) between 1996 and 2004 examined the use of acupuncture for symptom management mostly related to pain. Nearly 400 RCT results are reported in Medline for the same time period. Alrhough there is no evidence of the physical existence of *qi* or meridians, the effects of acupuncture are reportedly better than placebo in most trials [47]. Research has repeatedly and consistently demonstrated that opioid peptides, serotonin, and other neurotransmitters are released by acupuncture. Conclusive evidence has existed for some time that acupuncture is effective in the treatment of dental pain and postoperative nausea [44–48]. Efficacy of acupuncture in relief from asthma, back pain, drug dependency, fibromyalgia, migraine and tension headaches, neck pain, osteoarthritis, and stroke is considered inconclusive by some authors [47]. Others suggest the evidence is equivocal or promising for some indications such as addiction, stroke rehabilitation, postoperative- and chemotherapy-related nausea and vomiting, tennis elbow, carpal tunnel syndrome, and asthma [44–49].

Contraindications

"Needling" technique is contraindicated in patients with severe bleeding disorders or who are at increased risk for infection, such as patients who have neutropenia, women who are in the first trimester of pregnancy, with the exception of treatment for nausea, and patients who have cardiac pacemakers, who should not be treated with electrical stimulation [49,50]. Caution is advised for the first treatment, and some authors recommend that this treatment be administered with the patient in the supine position. Some patients become drowsy, and care should be taken regarding operating machinery, including driving. Needles should not be re-used and strict asepsis is mandatory [50]. Side effects include bleeding, bruising, pain with needling, and worsening of symptoms. Reported adverse events are rare but include pneumothorax and death [50].

Opportunities

Ernst [51] suggests that because the diagnostic value of acupuncture has not been established, it may constitute more risk than reward but that it is worthy of consideration for any number of conditions. There is evidence that with accurate diagnosis it is safe, and for certain conditions it is more effective than placebo when administered by an appropriately trained practitioner.

Examples of clinical trials

These three trials are examples of clinical trials: (1) phase III randomized study of acupressure for chemotherapy-induced nausea in women with breast cancer receiving one of three combination therapy regimens (MDA-NURO1-396); (2) randomized study of electroacupuncture for treatment of delayed chemotherapy-induced nausea and vomiting in patients with newly diagnosed pediatric sarcomas (NCCAM-02-AT-0172); and (3) randomized study of acupuncture to improve end-of-life symptom distress with patients with metastatic colorectal cancer (UPITTS-010,901).

Nationally, acupuncturists can be certified in various ways: (1) complete a formal, full-time educational program that includes classroom and clinical hours or (2) participate in an apprenticeship program. Physicians with training in acupuncture also may obtain board certification. All acupuncturists must also complete a "clean needle technique" approved course. The National Certification Commission of Acupuncture and Oriental Medicine established standards for certification accepted by some states for licensure. Physicians must possess a valid medical license and be certified through the American Academy of Medical Acupuncture (www.medicalacupuncture.org). A comparison of license versus certified acupuncturists can be accessed at a state professional licensure Web site.

Reiki

Reiki is an ancient form of healing that means "universal life energy." The practitioner acts as a conduit for the movement of energy. Reiki differs from other healing systems in that it is the energy—not the healer—that influences healing. That is, energy travels through the healing, not from the healer. Reiki is thought to alleviate physical, emotional, and spiritual blockages [52]. There are five premises of Reiki, (1) there is an energy of unique properties applicable to physical and psychologic conditions, (2) the energy has a source, (3) this source can be tapped, (4) a person can be taught to use this energy, and (5) the effects of this energy is palpable and subjective. The energy is not influenced by the practitioner's faith or religion and is considered pure [52]. The practitioner gently places his or her hands on the client in 12 specific positions for approximately 5 minutes per position, depending on the needs of the client. No pressure, massage, or manipulation is applied to the client, who remains clothed.

Highlights of evidence

Two MA examining Reiki (with therapeutic touch) were reported between 1999 and 2004. More than 20 RCTs are reported in Medline for 1999 to 2005. Reiki may be helpful in the treatment of pain, mood changes, and fatigue [53–55].

Contraindications

There are no known contraindications for Reiki [51].

Opportunities

Reiki seems to have few adverse effects and eventually can be self-administered.

Example of clinical trials

Reiki/Energy Healing in Prostate Cancer NCCAM, R21AT1120.

Practitioners

Typically, Reiki is taught in three parts. Reiki Part 1 includes history of Reiki, Reiki hand positions, and Reiki symbols and their meditation manifestation. Reiki II involves intense training focusing on advanced techniques and includes a review of Reiki I. The training for Reiki II brings knowledge of long distance healing, scanning techniques, and the long distance Reiki symbols and their names. Typically there are two USUI-REIKI-Tibetan attunements at intervals throughout the course. Reiki III (Master) includes a review of previous training and practice and brings to the student knowledge for long distance healing, scanning techniques, more meditation techniques, and an additional Reiki symbol. Typically, there is a Reiki attunement at the end of the course. There is no licensure for Reiki.

Herbal products

Herbal products were not regulated before the Dietary Supplement Health and Education Act (DSHEA) of 1994. As a result of this act, a dietary supplement is defined as a product intended to supplement the diet that may be a vitamin, mineral, herb, botanical, amino acid, a concentrate, metabolite, constituent, extract, supplement to increase total daily intake, or combination of these ingredients [56]. The product must be intended for ingestion in pill, capsule, tablet, or liquid form, must not be a conventional food or the sole item of a meal or diet, and must be labeled as a dietary supplement. The DSHEA provides for the use of various statements on a product label that do not need preapproval, although claims must not be made about the diagnosis, prevention, treatment, or cure for a specific disease. For example, a claim for an herb or supplement cannot read: "This product will cure breast cancer, heart disease, obesity and acne."

Dietary supplements must bear ingredient labeling (including name and quantity of each ingredient) and nutrition labeling (daily consumption recommendations). Botanical and herbal products must state the part of the plant from which the ingredient originated. DHSEA provides the US Food and Drug Administration the authority to develop good manufacturing practices governing all aspects of preparation, packing, and storing. The NIH Office of Dietary Supplements was created, through DSHEA, to promote, collect, and compile research and maintain a database on supplements and individual nutrients [57]. From a consumer standpoint, the DHSEA provides for over-the-counter, ready access to a wide range of products without the requirement of standardization [58].

Shark and bovine cartilage

Description

Also known as Arthrelan, Carticin, and Haifischknorpel, shark cartilage is derived from the fin of the hammerhead and spiny dogfish sharks. It was thought that shark cartilage might have anticancer properties because sharks did not seem to get cancer [59]. Some believe that creative marketing, not science, promoted this hypothesis [47]. Chemical ingredients include glycoproteins sphyrnastatin 1 and sphyrnastatin 2. Cartilage accounts for 6% of a shark's total body weight. Bovine (cow) cartilage and shark cartilage have been studied as cancer treatment for more than 30 years, and numerous products are sold as dietary supplements. Mechanisms of action have been proposed to explain the potential antitumor activity of cartilage: (1) direct cell kill, (2) immune system stimulation, and (3) angiogenesis. Three different angiogenesis inhibitors are identified in bovine cartilage, and two have been purified from shark cartilage [60].

Highlights of evidence

No MR or SA evaluating shark or bovine cartilage was reported through 2006. Seven RCTs (in vitro and in vivo) are reported in Medline for various conditions between 1995 and 2006. Few human studies of cartilage have been published, and results are considered inconclusive [60]. In animal studies, cartilage products have been administered by oral, injection, topical, and surgically implanted routes. Effects of cartilage on angiogenesis have been studied in chicken embryos, rabbit corneas, and mice conjunctiva [61]. In human studies, cartilage products have been administered via oral, topical, enema or subcutaneous injection route. The oral route of administration has caused challenges in trial design because human intestines do not allow the absorption of large molecules (sphyrnastatin) in quantities considered adequate for therapeutic benefit [62]. The dosage and duration of cartilage treatment has varied due to the different products used in trials. To date investigational new drug status has been granted to four groups of investigators to study cartilage as cancer treatment.

Contraindications

There are significant differences in commercially available cartilage products and purity. There are reported cases of hepatitis caused by shark cartilage [63]. Shark cartilage is contraindicated during pregnancy and lactation [64].

Example of clinical trials

The following clinical trial was conducted: phase III randomized study of induction platinum-based chemotherapy and radiotherapy with or without Æ-941 (Neovastat) in patients with unresectable stage IIIA or IIIB non-small cell lung cancer (MDA-ID-99,303, NCCAM, NCI-T99-0046).

Antioxidants

Antioxidant vitamins E, C, and beta-carotene and CoQ10 (Coenzyme Q 10, ubiquinone), which is an antioxidant found in all living cells, are believed to have powerful antioxidant effects. Although data are incomplete, it is reported that up to 30% of Americans are taking some form of antioxidant supplement. Researchers have shown that patients with cancer take antioxidants, typically at doses higher than recommended [65,66]. An antioxidant frequently used by patients with cancer is vitamin C. Ongoing debate surrounds antioxidants and cancer therapies. This debate includes the precept that cancer therapies create free radicals through their cytotoxic mechanism and antioxidants may interfere with this mechanism. Cancer therapies included in this debate include alkylating agents, antimetabolites, and radiation therapy. Limited research has supported the theory that chemotherapy diminishes total antioxidant status, but there have been difficulties and inconsistencies with research design preventing formulation of conclusions [66,67].

Highlights of evidence

More than 45 MR or SR reviewing antioxidants (of which 5 involve patients with cancer) are reported between 1994 and 2006. More than 2000 RCTs involving antioxidants are reported in Medline during this same time period. Concern that antioxidants may interfere with the efficacy of cancer therapy is not new. The association between beta carotene and increased risk of lung cancer in smokers is well known [68,69]. Conversely, some researchers have suggested that selective inhibition of tumor cell growth is an action of antioxidants, antioxidants may promote cellular differentiation with enhanced cytotoxic effects, and the dose of the antioxidant can determine efficacy [66,70,71]. Ray and colleagues [71] suggested that typically recommended doses may be insufficient to cover the higher production of reactive oxygen metabolites. Researchers have been concerned that although some antioxidants may decrease some kinds of toxicity associated with cancer chemotherapy, the therapeutic benefit of the cancer therapy may be compromised [66]. Ladas and colleagues reviewed more than 100 citations on antioxidant status and cancer outcomes and antioxidant use among patients receiving chemotherapy with or without radiation therapy. Of the 52 that met their research criteria, 31 were observational studies and 21 were intervention trials. Their findings showed a decline in the total antioxidant status of patients receiving cancer therapy but conflicting and inconsistent results regarding the effect of chemotherapy on antioxidant status in patients receiving cancer therapy [66,70,72]. Variability in doses, duration of supplementation, and timing of interventions have prevented the formulation of recommendations and conclusions [66,73].

Contraindications

Contraindications for specific antioxidants are related to those known (eg, beta carotene) and lung cancer risk among smokers. (1) Vitamin C: potential interactions may occur with aluminum antacids, cyclosporine, statins, calcium channel blockers and protease inhibitors, iron, and vitamin E [64]; (2) Vitamin E: potential interactions may occur with cholestramine, colestipol, mineral oil, anticonvulsants, anticoagulants, and verapamil [64]; (3) Beta-carotene: potential interactions may occur with cholestyramine, colestipol, mineral oil, and orlistat [64].

Example of clinical trials

The following trial was conducted: phase III randomized study of selenium and vitamin E for the prevention of prostate cancer (SELECT Trial), NCCAM, NCI, SWOG-S0000.

Practitioners

Registered dieticians have a minimum of a bachelors degree in dietetics. Certified nutritionists have education and training in clinical nutrition and may be a nurse or other health care professional. Caution should be taken when choosing nutrition practitioners to ensure that they have expertise in oncology and supplements and nutrition.

Symptom management

Patients use CAM for cancer treatment and symptom management. Symptom management in cancer care begins at the time of diagnosis and continues through survivorship. Remarkable advances have been made in minor to major aspects of symptom management associated with cancer, its treatment, and long-term consequences of both. Oncology nurses are experts in cancer symptom management by reducing the overall impact of symptoms on health outcomes [74]. Quality cancer care, as identified by the Oncology Nursing Society, supports appropriate symptom management as a supportive care component [75]. The current Putting Evidence into Practice resources include the Priority Symptom Management (PRISM) project developed by the ONS Foundation Center for Leadership, Information, and Research in 2000, which focusin on six primary symptoms: anorexia, cognitive dysfunction, depression, fatigue, neutropenia, and pain [37]. Although there is limited decisive evaluation of the quality of CAM approaches in symptom management, patients continue to use CAM therapies alone or with conventional approaches to manage symptoms.

Anorexia

Anorexia is defined as the loss of the compensatory increase in feeding. Anorexia, involuntary weight loss, tissue wasting, poor performance, and ultimately death characterize the condition of advanced protein calorie malnutrition, also referred to as cachexia [76,77]. The cancer anorexia-cachexia syndrome is a maladaptive, multidimensional process involving physiologic and behavioral components that correlate with compromised quality of life and poor outcomes. Abnormalities in the mouth and digestive tract (dysphagia, odynophagia, early satiety, erosive lesions), changes in taste and smell, learned aversion to specific foods, and cancer treatment (effects of chemotherapy and radiation therapy) contribute to this syndrome. Conventional approaches for anorexia/cachexia include (1) curing the cancer, (2) increasing nutritional intake, (3) inhibiting muscle and fat wasting, and (4) identifying the causes of reduced food intake. Conventional interventions include glucocorticoids and progesterones, cannabinoids, antiserotonergic drugs, and metoclopramide. CAM modalities have included melatonin and hydrazine sulfate. In early studies using melatonin, a loss of more than 10% body weight was less common among patients treated with melatonin compared with placebo [78,79]. Later studies were less conclusive [64,80,81]. Inhibition of phosphoenolpyruvate carboxykinase was seen with the use of hydrazine sulfate. There was no normalization of carbohydrate metabolism reported in anorectic/cachectic cancer patients in early studies. Later research did not demonstrate any benefit [64,82,83].

A role for oncology nurses in cancer complementary and alternative medicine

Given the sustained use of CAM therapies, oncology nurses must become knowledgeable in understanding the role of CAM in cancer care. A model for cancer CAM care begins with the transdisciplinary team: (1) clarifying fact from fiction, (2) acknowledging misperceptions about CAM, and (3) mixing and unmixing therapies [83]. A baseline knowledge of CAM beginning with evaluating personal and professional beliefs is mandatory [3]. Nurses can begin peer education and establish standards of practice in CAM therapy delivery across practice settings once they are knowledgeable about evidence-based safe and effective use of these therapies. Nurses must ensure that practitioners with proper training deliver CAM therapies and

Box 2. Endpoints for the role of nursing in cancer complementary and alternative medicine

Expand individual baseline knowledge regarding cancer CAM through oral and written modes and experiential learning

Provide high-quality patient and peer education regarding safety and efficacy of CAM therapies

Facilitate partnerships among patients, conventional HCP, CAM providers, and colleagues to discuss knowledge and perspective about cancer CAM

Seek proper training, demonstrate competency, and obtain necessary credentials if practicing a CAM therapy

Request and require informed consent (with witness) of patients receiving a CAM therapy

Ensure proper credentialing of a CAM provider before recommending provider to patients

Establish institutional-specific standards of practice for the use of CAM therapies within specific patient populations

Document patient consent procedures, tolerance, and response to CAM therapy

Design a new or assist in the quality maintenance of a pre-established integrative care program

Develop and update a working knowledge of cost issues and reimbursement of CAM in the community

Collaborate in the design of methodologically rigorous cancer CAM treatment and supportive care clinical trials

Contribute to the body of nursing knowledge in cancer CAM through publications and presentations in the United States and internationally

---

From Decker G, Lee C. Complementary and alternative medicine (CAM) therapies. In: Yarbro C, Frogge M, Goodman M, editors. Cancer nursing principles and practice. 6th edition. Sudbury (MA): Jones and Bartlett; 2005. p. 613; with permission.

ensure that patients sign informed consent. The medical record must contain documentation of the consent procedures, tolerance, and response to CAM therapy [84,85]. Major endpoints for the role of nursing in cancer CAM are offered by Lee and are seen in Box 2.

References

[1] Whorton JC. The history of complementary and alternative medicine. In: Jonas WB, Levin JS, editors. Essentials complementary and alternative medicine. Philadelphia: Lippincott Williams & Wilkins; 1999.

[2] National Cancer Institute. Cancer facts: complementary and alternative medicine in cancer treatment: questions and answers. Fact Sheet 9.14. 2003.
[3] Oncology Nursing Society Position. The use of complementary and alternative therapies in cancer care. Pittsburgh (PA): Oncology Nursing Society; 2006.
[4] Decker G, Lee C. Complementary and alternative medicine (CAM) therapies. In: Yarbro C, Frogge M, Goodman M, editors. Cancer nursing principles and practice. 6th edition. Sudbury (MA): Jones and Bartlett; 2005. p. 590–620.
[5] White JD. Complementary and alternative medicine research: a National Cancer Institute perspective. Semin Oncol 2002;29(6):546–51.
[6] Antman K, Benson M, Chabot J, et al. Complementary and alternative medicine: the role of the cancer center. J Clin Oncol 2001;19(18 Suppl):55S–60S.
[7] Furnham A. Why do people choose and use complementary therapies? In: Ernst E, editor. Complementary medicine: an objective appraisal. Oxford (MS): Butterworth Heinemann; 1996. p. 71–88.
[8] Kaptchuk TJ, Eisenberg DM. The persuasive appeal of alternative medicine. Ann Intern Med 1998;129(12):1061–5.
[9] Kessler RC, Davis R, Foster D, et al. Long-term trends in the use of complementary and alternative medical therapies in the United States. Ann Intern Med 2001;135(4):262–8.
[10] National Center for Complementary and Alternative Medicine. 2004. Available at: http://nccam.nih.gov/. Accessed September 17, 2007.
[11] Office of cancer complementary and alternative medicine. 2004. National Cancer Institute. Available at: http://www.cancer.gov/cam/. Accessed September 17, 2007.
[12] White J. Cancer: current research in alternative therapies. Primary Care Clinics in Office Practice 29(2):379–92.
[13] White House Commission on Complementary and Alternative Medicine. March 2002. Final report. Available at: www.whccamp.hhs.gov. Accessed September 17, 2007.
[14] Institutes of Medicine. Use of complementary and alternative medicine (CAM) by the American public. Available at: www.iom.edu/CMS/3793/4829.aspx. Accessed September 17, 2007.
[15] Stevinson C. Why patients use complementary and alternative medicine. In: Ernst E, editor. The desktop guide to complementary and alternative medicine: an evidence-based approach. Edinburg (TX): Harcourt Publishers Limited; 2001. p. 395–403.
[16] National Center for Complementary and Alternative Medicine. The use of complementary and alternative medicine in the United States. Available at: http://nccam.nih.gov/news/camsurvey_fs1.htm. Accessed November 19, 2007.
[17] Berk LB. Primer on Integrative Oncology. Hematol Oncol Clin North Am 2006;213–31.
[18] Eisenberg DM, Kessler R, Foster C, et al. Unconventional medicine in the United States: prevalence, costs, and patterns of use. N Engl J Med 1993;328(4):246–52.
[19] Eisenberg DM, Davuis RB, Ettner SR, et al. Trends in alternative medicine use in the United States, 1990–1997: results of a follow-up national survey. JAMA 1998;280(18):1569–75.
[20] Basch E, Ulbricht C. Prevalence of CAM use among US cancer patients: an update. Journal of Cancer Integrative Medicine 2004;2(1):13–4.
[21] Ni H, Simile C, Hardy AM. Utilization of complementary and alternative medicine by United States adults: results from the 1999 national health interview survey. Med Care 2002;40(4):353–8.
[22] Ernst E, Cassileth BR. The prevalence of complementary/alternative medicine in cancer: a systematic review. Cancer 1998;83(4):777–82.
[23] Bennett M, Lengacher C. Use of complementary therapies in a rural cancer population. Oncol Nurs Forum 1999;26(8):1287–94.
[24] Sparber A, Wootton JC, Bauer L, et al. Use of complementary medicine by adult patients participating in cancer clinical trials. Oncol Nurs Forum 2000;27(4):623–30.
[25] Bernstein BJ, Grasso T. Prevalence of complementary and alternative medicine use in cancer patients. Oncology (Huntingt) 2001;15(10):1267–72 [discussion: 1272–8, 1283].

[26] Vallerand AH, Fouladbakhsh JM, Templin T. The use of complementary/alternative medicine therapies for the self-treatment of pain among residents of urban, suburban, and rural communities. Am J Public Health 2003;93(6):923–5.
[27] Najm W, Reinsch S, Hoehler F, et al. Use of complementary and alternative medicine among the ethnic elderly. Altern Ther Health Med 2003;9(3):50–7.
[28] Herron M, Glasser M. Use of and attitudes toward complementary and alternative medicine among family practice patients in small rural Illinois communities. J Rural Health 2003; 19(3):279–84.
[29] Ashikaga T, Bosompra K, O'Brien P, et al. Use of complimentary and alternative medicine by breast cancer patients: prevalence, patterns and communication with physicians. Support Care Cancer 2002;10(7):542–8.
[30] Maskarinec G, Shumay DM, Kakai H, et al. Ethnic differences in complementary and alternative medicine use among cancer patients. J Altern Complement Med 2000;6(6):531–8.
[31] Richardson MA, Sanders T, Palmer JL, et al. Complementary/alternative medicine use in a comprehensive cancer center and the implications for oncology. J Clin Oncol 2000; 18(13):2505–14.
[32] Swisher EM, Cohn DE, Goff BA, et al. Use of complementary and alternative medicine among women with gynecologic cancers. Gynecol Oncol 2002;84(3):363–7.
[33] Lengacher CA, Bennett MP, Kipp K, et al. Design and testing of the use of a complementary and alternative therapies survey in women with breast cancer. Oncol Nurs Forum 2003; 30(5):811–21.
[34] Bridevaux IP. A survey of patients' out-of-pocket payments for complementary and alternative medicine therapies. Complement Ther Med 2004;12(1):48–50.
[35] White A. Economic issues in complementary and alternative medicine. In: Ernst E, editor. The desktop guide to complementary and alternative medicine. Edinburgh: Mosby; 2001. p. 415–22.
[36] Oxford Centre for Evidence-based Medicine. Headington, Oxford: University Department of Psychiatry, Warneford Hospital; 2004. Available at: www.cebm.net.
[37] Natural Standard. Natural Standard database. University of Texas M.D. Anderson Cancer Center. 2004.
[38] Natural medicines comprehensive database. 2004. Available at: www.naturaldatabase.com. Accessed September 17, 2007.
[39] PRISM Project—ONS Foundation—now available at PEP Resource Center. Available at: www.ons.org/research/information/documents/pdfs/ONSResAgendaFinal10-24-07.pdf. Accessed October 3, 2007.
[40] Hilsden RJ, Verhoef MJ. Complementary therapies: evaluating their effectiveness in cancer. Patient Educ Couns 1999;38(2):101–8.
[41] Pelletier K. The best alternative medicine. New York: Simon & Schuster; 2007.
[42] Long AF. Outcome measurement in complementary and alternative medicine: unpicking the effects. J Altern Complement Med 2002;8(6):777–86.
[43] Mayer DJ. Acupuncture: an evidence-based review of the clinical literature. Annu Rev Med 2000;51:49–63.
[44] MacPherson H, Schroera S. Acupuncture as a complex intervention for depression: a consensus method to develop a standardised treatment protocol for a randomised controlled trial. Complement Ther Med 2007;15:92–100.
[45] Ernst E, Pittler MH. The effectiveness of acupuncture in treating acute dental pain: a systematic review. Br Dent J 1998;184(9):443–7.
[46] Vickers AJ. Can acupuncture have specific effects on health? A systematic review of acupuncture antiemesis trials. J R Soc Med 1996;89(6):303–11.
[47] Melchart D, Linde K, Fisher P, et al. Acupuncture for recurrent headaches: a systematic review of randomized controlled trials. Cephalalgia 1999;19(9):779–86 [discussion: 765].
[48] Han JS, Terenius L. Neurochemical basis of acupuncture analgesia. Annu Rev Pharmacol Toxicol 1982;22:193–220.

[49] Aikins Murphy P. Alternative therapies for nausea and vomiting of pregnancy. Obstet Gynecol 1998;91(1):149–55.
[50] Ernst E, White A. Life-threatening adverse reactions after acupuncture? A systematic review. Pain 1997;71(2):123–6.
[51] Ernst E, editor. The desktop guide to complementary and alternative medicine: an evidence-based approach. London (UK): Mosby; 2001.
[52] Segen JC. Dictionary of alternative medicine. Stamford (CT): Appleton & Lange; 1998.
[53] Olson K, Hanson J. Using Reiki to manage pain: a preliminary report. Cancer Prev Control 1997;1(2):108–13.
[54] Lafreniere KD, et al. Effects of therapeutic touch on biochemical and mood indicators in women. J Altern Complement Med 1999;5(4):367–70.
[55] Post-White J, Kinney ME, Savik K, et al. Therapeutic massage and healing touch improve symptoms in cancer. Integr Cancer Ther 2003;2(4):332–44.
[56] Dietary Supplement Health and Education Act of 1994. Public Law 103–417. 1994.
[57] Office of Dietary Supplements. Bethesda (MD): National Institutes of Health; 2004. Available at: http://ods.od.nih.gov/.
[58] Kinsel JF, Straus SE. Complementary and alternative therapeutics: rigorous research is needed to support claims. Annu Rev Pharmacol Toxicol 2003;43:463–84 [epub 2002 Jan 10].
[59] Lane IW, Comac L. Sharks don't get cancer. Garden City Park (NY): Avery Publishing Group, Inc; 1992.
[60] PDQ®. PDQ® cancer information summaries: complementary and alternative medicine. Available at: www.nci.nih.gov/cancertopics/pdq/CAM. Accessed September 17, 2007.
[61] Gonzalez RP, Soares FS, Farids RF, et al. Demonstration of inhibitory effect of oral shark cartilage on basic fibroblast growth factor-induced angiogenesis in the rabbit cornea. Biol Pharm Bull 2001;24(2):151–4.
[62] Miller DR, Anderson, Stark, et al. Phase I/II trial of the safety and efficacy of shark cartilage in the treatment of advanced cancer. J Clin Oncol 1998;16(11):3649–55.
[63] Gotay CC, Dumitriu D. Health food store recommendations for breast cancer patients. Arch Fam Med 2000;9(8):692–9.
[64] PDR. PDR for nutritional supplements. Montvale (NJ): Medical Economics Company; 2001.
[65] VandeCreek L, Rogers E, Lester J. Use of alternative therapies among breast cancer outpatients compared with the general population. Altern Ther Health Med 1999;5(1):71–6.
[66] Ladas EJ, Jacobson JS, Kennedy DD, et al. Antioxidants and cancer therapy: a systematic review. J Clin Oncol 2004;22(3):517–28.
[67] Durken M, Herrnring C, Finckh B, et al. Impaired plasma antioxidative defense and increased nontransferrin-bound iron during high-dose chemotherapy and radiochemotherapy preceding bone marrow transplantation. Free Radic Biol Med 2000;28(6):887–94.
[68] Omenn GS, Goodman GE, Thornquist MD, et al. Effects of a combination of beta carotene and vitamin A on lung cancer and cardiovascular disease. N Engl J Med 1996;334(18): 1150–5.
[69] Albanes D, Heinones OP, Huttunen JK, et al. Effects of alpha-tocopherol and beta-carotene supplements on cancer incidence in the Alpha-Tocopherol Beta-Carotene Cancer Prevention Study. Am J Clin Nutr 1995;62(Suppl 6):1427S–30S.
[70] Conklin KA. Dietary antioxidants during cancer chemotherapy: impact on chemotherapeutic effectiveness and development of side effects. Nutr Cancer 2000;37(1):1–18.
[71] Ray SD, Patel D, Wong V, et al. In vivo protection of DNA damage associated apoptotic and necrotic cell deaths during acetaminophen-induced nephrotoxicity, amiodarone-induced lung toxicity and doxorubicin-induced cardiotoxicity by a novel IH636 grape seed proanthocyanidin extract. Res Commun Mol Pathol Pharmacol 2000;107(1–2):137–66.

[72] Jonas CR, Puckett AB, Jones JP, et al. Plasma antioxidant status after high-dose chemotherapy: a randomized trial of parenteral nutrition in bone marrow transplantation patients. Am J Clin Nutr 2000;72(1):181–9.
[73] Food and Nutrition Board. IOM Food and Nutrition Board. 2006. Available at: http://www.iom.edu/CMS/. Accessed September 17, 2007.
[74] Ropka ME, Spencer-Cisek P. PRISM: priority Symptom Management Project phase I: assessment. Oncol Nurs Forum 2001;28(10):1585–94.
[75] Oncology Nursing Society. Quality cancer care (Oncology Nursing Society position statement). Pittsburgh (PA): Oncology Nursing Society; 2000.
[76] Inui A. Cancer anorexia-cachexia syndrome: current issues in research and management. CA Cancer J Clin 2002;52(2):72–91.
[77] Inui A, Meguid MM. Cachexia and obesity: two sides of one coin? Curr Opin Clin Nutr Metab Care 2003;6(4):395–9.
[78] Lissoni P, Paolorossi F, Yanconi G, et al. Is there a role for melatonin in the treatment of neoplastic cachexia? Eur J Cancer 1996;32A(8):1340–3.
[79] Lissoni P. Is there a role for melatonin in supportive care? Suppor Cancer Care 2002;10(2):110–6.
[80] Mantovani G, Maccio A, Massa E, et al. Managing cancer-related anorexia/cachexia. Drugs 2001;61(4):499–514.
[81] Lee C. Complementary and alternative medicines patients are talking about: melatonin. Clin J Oncol Nurs 2006;10(1):105–7.
[82] Loprinzi CL, Goldberg RM, Su JQ, et al. Placebo-controlled trial of hydrazine sulfate in patients with newly diagnosed non-small-cell lung cancer. J Clin Oncol 1994;12(6):1126–9.
[83] Loprinzi CL, Kuross SA, O'Fallon JR, et al. Randomized placebo-controlled evaluation of hydrazine sulfate in patients with advanced colorectal cancer. J Clin Oncol 1994;12(6):1121–5.
[84] Lee CO. CAM in the 21st century in the US: role of nursing and evidence-based practice efforts. Presented at the 4th Annual Oncology Nursing Society Institutes of Learning. Philadelphia, PA; November 2003.
[85] Lee C. Clinical trials in cancer part I: biomedical, complementary, and Alternative Medicine: finding active trials and results of closed trials. Clin J Oncol Nurs 2004;8(5):531–5.

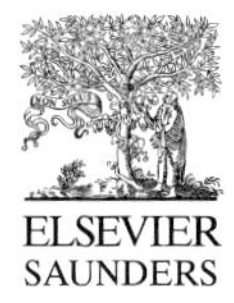
ELSEVIER
SAUNDERS

Nurs Clin N Am 43 (2008) 243–258

NURSING
CLINICS
OF NORTH AMERICA

The Changing Legacy of Cancer: Issues of Long-Term Survivorship

Susan A. Leigh, BSN, RN

National Coalition for Cancer Survivorship, 5050 East Golder Ranch Drive, Tucson, AZ 85739, USA

> *Day-by-day survivorship is a victory because it is the act of living on, no matter what happens.*
>
> Fitzhugh Mullan [1]

It has been approximately 2 decades since advocates created a new social movement by teaming the concept of survivorship with cancer. Surely this seemed like an oxymoron within a society that generally equated cancer with death. In *Illness as Metaphor*, Susan Sontag [2] wrote about the fear surrounding cancer and the general belief that "if it was not fatal, it was not cancer." But times were changing, and patients and family members who were affected by this disease identified the need for new terminology to describe the experience of living with, through, and beyond cancer [3]. Not only were patients living longer with new types of treatment but also there were guarded whispers about the possibility of cure. A newfound sense of hope was on the rise. Yet there were concerns about the complexities of surviving cancer, about healing body and spirit, about learning to live with leftover trauma—this truly was uncharted territory. This was survivorship. As Dr. Mullan [1] wrote, this was the "challenge faced daily by millions of Americans who are engaged in defiance of disease and in affirmation of life."

Historical evolution of survivorship

> *Arguably, without substantial numbers of survivors, issues of "survivorship" would never have become of interest; the focus of research would have remained, as it had in the past, largely on trying simply to enable an individual to become a survivor, not what the future of that person's life might be like.*
>
> Julia Rowland, Office of Cancer Survivorship [4]

E-mail address: sleigh@mindspring.com

doi:10.1016/j.cnur.2008.02.002 *nursing.theclinics.com*

When the War on Cancer first was declared in 1971, there were approximately 3 million survivors in the United States. Current estimates show close to 11 million cancer survivors in this country alone and almost 25 million worldwide [4,5]. These numbers reflect anyone who has a history of cancer, from those newly diagnosed to long-term survivors, including the terminally ill. In addition to the above numbers,

- Approximately 80% of children treated for cancer can expect to live for at least 5 years, whereas survivors under the age of 19 now have a 10-year survival approaching 75% [6].
- The 5-year survival estimate for adults is up to 64% with approximately 14% diagnosed more than 20 years ago [6].
- Three out of every four American families have at least one family member diagnosed with cancer [7].
- One of six persons over age 65 is living with a history of cancer [5].

Although these numbers reflect the many successes in science, technology, early detection, treatment developments, and care delivery, they also reveal a new set of challenges. These challenges include lingering and late effects of treatment and include questions about who will care for this growing population and who will pay the added costs. But first, let us take a look at how we got here.

Many in the medical community think of survivorship as a new field of research, care, and responsibility, especially since the recent release of the Institute of Medicine (IOM) report, *From Cancer Patient to Cancer Survivor: Lost in Transition* [8]. Yet, the evolution of this movement to increased awareness about survivorship has been going on for more than 20 years (Table 1).

While the Beatles were turning the musical world upside down in the 1960s, a quiet transformation was taking place in the medical world. New drug combinations were introduced to treat certain types of cancer. Cobalt treatments were being replaced by linear accelerators. Dr. Elizabeth Kubler-Ross brought the topic of death and dying out of the closet. Patients rarely had been told that they had cancer as this was considered an automatic death sentence. But times were changing.

By the time the 1970s began, the new specialty of oncology emerged to join the discipline of hematology. Whereas hematologists treated patients who had malignancies of blood and blood-forming tissues, oncologists specialized in the treatment of solid tumors. In December of 1971, President Nixon was persuaded to declare the War on Cancer by signing the National Cancer Act, and many believed that the magic bullet to cure cancer would soon be found. Patients were treated in cancer clinics or oncology wards, and it was almost impossible for anyone to not know their diagnosis. Nurses also recognized the need to specialize as they attempted to find ways to deliver chemotherapy safely, treat the debilitating side effects from drugs and radiation, and help support patients and their loved ones through the

Table 1
Evolution of survivorship

1960s	Development of clinical trials in cancer began to show promise, especially in pediatrics Diagnosis of cancer withheld from most patients Dr. Kubler-Ross talked openly about death and dying
1970s	Most patients told of their cancer diagnosis National Cancer Act signed by President Nixon 5-Year survival identified as measure of success
1980s	Support groups, community resource centers, and consumer publications focused on quality-of-life issues Field of psycho-oncology emerged Concept of survivorship introduced by NCCS (1986)
1990s	Disease-specific advocacy exploded into multiple organizations NCCS released *Imperatives for Cancer Care* (1995) OCS established at NCI (1996) THE MARCH on Washington (1998)
2000s	Plethora of government reports included survivorship issues • 2003: Childhood Cancer Survivorship: Improving Care and Quality of Life (IOM) • 2003: Living Beyond Cancer: Finding a New Balance (President's Cancer Panel) • 2004: A National Action Plan for Cancer Survivorship: Advancing Public Health Strategies (CDC, LAF) • 2005–2006: From Cancer Patient to Cancer Survivor: Lost in Transition (IOM) • 2007: Cancer Care for the Whole Patient: Meeting Psychosocial Health Needs (IOM)

grueling treatments [9]. Also, successful treatments for some pediatric cancers were found, and any child who lived for 5 years without a recurrence of disease was called a survivor. Success was measured in the number of months or years that patients survived—in other words, physical survival. But some parents began to wonder if treatment at any cost was really worth all the pain and suffering as they realized that surviving was more than just being alive.

By the 1980s, increasing numbers of patients who had cancer were living longer with a new, if tentative, sense of hope. Trial-and-error survival became the norm as there were no guidelines about what happens after treatment ends. Just as patients and their loved ones learned how to talk about dying from cancer, the topic soon progressed to living with cancer. Psycho-oncology became a formalized component of cancer-related research and care, and the semantics of survival were defined in broader strokes to reflect not only longevity but also the experience of surviving. As quality of life increased in importance, communities responded to these newly identified needs and started developing support groups, publications, networking opportunities, resource centers, and general cancer advocacy organizations.

With this increasing awareness about living with cancer, the 1990s saw the creation of new advocacy organizations that focused more specifically on individual diseases. Different breast cancer groups organized around education, support, research, clinical trials, fundraising, advocacy, causation, and environmental issues. Ovarian cancer advocates soon followed by establishing their own networks and adding their voices to the public policy arena. Men jumped on board and designed prostate cancer groups that included spouses or partners. Those who had multiple myeloma, lymphoma, leukemia, or colorectal, pancreatic, or lung cancer, separated into their own organizations. Consumer advocates no longer could be ignored as they organized, networked, marched, and raised their collective voices to be part of health care debates. Meanwhile, oncology nurses played major roles in advocating for patient rights, researching lingering and late effects, helping to develop patient-focused organizations, and raising awareness about survivorship issues.

With the 1995 release of the National Coalition for Cancer Survivorship (NCCS) report, *Imperatives for Quality Cancer Care: Access, Advocacy, Action & Accountability* [10], a new era of survivorship awareness was set into motion. The Director of the National Cancer Institute (NCI) at that time, Dr. Richard Klausner, read the report and asked why nothing was being done about these issues. Within 1 year, the Office of Cancer Survivorship (OCS) was established at NCI "in recognition of the growing population of cancer survivors and their unique and poorly understood needs" [11]. Box 1 describes the work of the OCS. Shortly after the creation of this important office, NCCS led an ambitious national grassroots campaign to make the cause, the care, and the cure of cancer the nation's top health priority, culminating in "THE MARCH…Coming Together to Conquer Cancer" [12]. Thus, the century ended having paved the way to a new era of cancer care.

Finally, survivorship was on the national agenda. As the new century was begun, many government reports were released that focused on survivorship issues:

- 2003—*Childhood Cancer Survivorship: Improving Care and Quality of Life*. From the IOM and National Research Council of the National Academy of Science [13]. Issues of long-term survival invariably were first identified in pediatrics.
- 2004—*Living Beyond Cancer: Finding a New Balance*. From the President's Cancer Panel [14]. Lance Armstrong sat as consumer advocate on this prestigious panel, offering high visibility to this report that differentiates survivor issues across the lifespan.
- 2004—*A National Action Plan for Cancer Survivorship: Advancing Public Health Strategies*. From Centers for Disease Control (CDC) and the Lance Armstrong Foundation (LAF) [15]. Looks at the burden of cancer as a public health issue and promotes culturally sensitive research and care.
- 2005 (introduced), 2006 (released)—*From Cancer Patient to Cancer Survivor: Lost in Transition*. From the IOM [8]. Surely this is the big bang of reports with a major focus on adult survivorship issues and the phase

Box 1. Office of cancer survivorship

- The OCS was established in 1996 by the NCI in recognition of the large number of individuals surviving cancer for long periods of time.
- The OCS is dedicated to enhancing the length and quality of life of more than 10 million cancer survivors in the United States and addressing their unique and poorly understood needs.
- The OCS considers individuals survivors from the time of diagnosis through the balance of their lives. Because friends, family members, and caregivers also are affected by a cancer diagnosis, they are included in this definition.
- The OCS supports and promotes research that examines and addresses the long- and short-term effects of cancer and its treatment. These include physical, psychologic, social, and economic effects among pediatric and adult survivors and their families. Survivorship research focuses on the physical, emotional, social, and financial outcomes beyond the treatment phase and seeks to optimize the health and well-being of persons living with a history of cancer. Survivorship research also seeks to provide a knowledge base regarding optimal follow-up care and surveillance of new or recurrent cancers.

of care that follows initial treatment. Builds on work of previous documents and offers 10 comprehensive recommendations (Box 2).

- 2007—*Cancer Care for the Whole Patient: Meeting Psychosocial Health Needs*. The latest report from the IOM that emphasizes how technology alone is not enough to deliver quality cancer care [16].

Now that survivorship and its plethora of issues can no longer be denied, just what are these issues? According to these reports, the healthcare community was not doing a very good job at identifying problems and taking care of survivors. But first, how is this population defined?

Defining population

Many articles, chapters, textbooks, Web sites, and conferences are devoted to issues surrounding cancer survivors and survivorship. Many are focused on educating oncology professionals and an equal number educate survivors and anyone in a supportive role. Although it is tempting to think that surviving a deadly disease should be reward enough, many survivors face complications, lingering and delayed, that cover a spectrum from mildly annoying to life threatening. But, first, what parameters define survivorship?

Box 2. From cancer patient to cancer survivor: lost in transition recommendations

1. Raise awareness.
2. Provide care plan.
3. Develop clinical practice guidelines.
4. Define quality health care.
5. Overcome delivery system challenges.
6. Include as public health concern.
7. Improve professional capacity.
8. Address employment-related concerns.
9. Improve access to health insurance.
10. Invest in research.

There is little agreement among oncology researchers, clinicians, caregivers, and patients themselves as to who is labeled a survivor and when. Is someone a patient when receiving treatment and a survivor when it is over? Must a patient wait 5 years and remain free of disease before this label can be applied? Is a patient a survivor from the moment of diagnosis and the remainder of life? Any and all of these labels are considered accurate depending on the context of the situation. Meanwhile, many survivors themselves loathe the term and identify themselves in any number of ways other than survivor: patient, veteran, victor, fighter, conqueror, sufferer, activist, warrior, thriver, or advocate. Rather than argue about who is right or wrong in defining this population, the concept of survivorship often is discussed. Although NCCS first introduced this concept as far back as 1986, there still is no consensus as to how this term is defined. It can be identified as a time frame, an outcome of treatment, a stage or phase, or a process of survival (Box 3). The easiest way to deal with the controversy is to dcfinc the terms depending on the program, project, or population being served.

Box 3. Defining survivorship

As a time frame: after 2, 5, or 10 years, depending on the type and stage of disease

As an outcome: no evidence of disease, complete remission, or cured

As a stage or phase: follows end of primary treatment and before another problem occurs

As a process: the dynamic experience of living through different stages of illness

Meanwhile, the population that is generating the most debate and needing attention is longer-term survivors who have completed an initial course of therapy. This is hardly, however, a homogeneous group. (Box 4 lists examples of the different paths survivors can take.)

Consequences of cancer

> *There had been no formal exit from sick to well, no instruction sheet on what to do next with my life. Cancer was my "trial by fire". In surviving it, I had learned many precious lessons. Perhaps one of the most important: Staying alive is just the initial challenge; living with the consequences of the disease and therapy becomes a lifelong responsibility* [17].

Box 4. Different survivorship paths

- Some survivors have completed treatment within the past few months or even the past few years, whereas others were treated decades ago.
- Some survivors recover from the effects of treatments with little difficulty and feel almost normal within a few short months, whereas other survivors take much more time to recuperate from the trauma of treatment.
- Some survivors live in "remission" whereas others are considered cured.
- Some survivors remain on maintenance therapy for months to years to keep the cancer or side effects under control.
- Some survivors live for many years with metastatic cancer with hopes that different treatment can control a disease considered incurable.
- Some survivors may experience a recurrence of their original cancer.
- Some survivors may be diagnosed with second malignancies.
- Some survivors may discover that their cancer treatments have damaged other parts of their bodies, such as their heart, ovaries, testes, or lungs.
- Some survivors recover physically but may have difficulty recovering from emotional or social fallout from treatment.
- And, finally, although many survivors recover physically, they may have difficulty recovering from emotional or social traumas that may be fallout from treatment and that often are more difficult for some survivors to deal with than the medical problems.

Consequences of cancer and its treatment can be categorized in several ways. Initially, they can be looked at as long-term (lingering or persistent) effects or late (delayed) effects. Both types of effects also can be considered aftereffects of treatment [18]. Lingering effects are chronic sequelae that persist after treatment ends and might include such physiologic side effects as post-treatment pain, fatigue, peripheral neuropathy, cognitive dysfunction, or endocrine imbalances. These particular symptoms also could be classified as late effects depending on the circumstances, such as surfacing months to years after treatment ends. More obvious examples of late physiologic effects are recurrence of original disease, development of secondary cancers, and organ system failures (Table 2).

Besides the physiologic sequelae, the cancer experience can have an impact on other domains of life. These often are equally, and sometimes more, affected than the physical domain and include psychologic (emotional), social (including vocational or financial), and spiritual (existential) domains. Volumes have been published about these distinct yet interconnected domains. Nurses, social workers, psychologists, physicians, and survivors themselves have identified, described, researched, and published

Table 2
Examples of physiologic sequelae

System specific
- Organ damage or failure
- Cardiac (eg, cardiomyopathy, coronary artery disease, or pericardial effusion)
- Pulmonary (eg, fibrosis or pneumonitis)
- Endocrine (eg, hypothyroidism, sterility, or premature menopause)
- Vascular (eg, stroke, arterial stenosis, transient ischemic attack, or avascular necrosis)
- Compromised immune system (eg, decreased immune function or increased risk for infection)

Second malignant neoplasms
- Recurrence of primary malignancy.
- Cancer associated with primary malignancy (eg, ovarian cancer after primary breast cancer)
- Cancer associated with past therapies (eg, breast cancer after chest irradiation)

Functional changes
- Decreased energy
- Incontinence
- Lymphedema
- Pain
- Neuropathies
- Fatigue
- Amputations
- Cataracts
- Dental caries

Cosmetic changes
- Lymphedema
- Amputations, including mastectomy
- Ostomies
- Weight gain and weight loss
- Skin or hair alterations

reports and studies about cancer survivorship. The recent IOM report, *Cancer Care for the Whole Patient: Meeting Psychosocial Health Needs,* states that "good quality health care must attend to patients' psychosocial problems and provide services to enable them to better manage their illnesses and underlying health. To ignore these factors while we pour billions of dollars into new technologies, is like spending all one's money on the latest model car and then not have the money left to buy the gas needed to make it run" [16].

Following are examples of other possible aftereffects identified by many researchers and cancer survivors [6,19–23].

- Psychologic aftereffects: fear of recurrence, chronic anxiety, uncertainty about future, fear of dependency, survivor guilt, post-traumatic stress disorder, depression, anger, concerns about body image
- Social aftereffects: change in social roles or relationships, distress within family unit, employment discrimination/problems, insurance and financial concerns
- Spiritual aftereffects: creating "new normal" or rediscovering self, questioning the meaning of illness and life after cancer, changing sense of hope and future, change in relationship with organized religion and God, surviving existential crisis and need to give back

Although sexual issues and sexuality often are included in one or more of these categories, a separate category illustrates the complexity of this domain:

- Sexuality aftereffects: can be a combination of physiologic, psychologic, social, or spiritual effects

Physiologic changes, such as vaginal atrophy or erectile dysfunction, can lead to psychologic distress. Psychologic distress, including depression, body image and self-esteem issues, can lead to social problems. Social problems, such as divorce, dating, or job loss, can affect a sense of self or existential being. Thus, aftereffects from cancer and treatment often are intertwined and difficult to separate into neat categories. This example also illustrates the increasingly popular mind-body-spirit connection. In the *State of the Science on Nursing Approaches to Managing Late and Long-Term Sequelae of Cancer and Cancer Treatment*, a special issue of the *American Journal of Nursing* (*AJN*), three articles covered issues surrounding the topic of sexuality: "Sexuality and Body Image," "Reproductive and Hormonal Sequelae of Chemotherapy in Women," and "Endocrine and Fertility Effects in Male Cancer Survivors" [23–26].

These aftereffects are so general that they only introduce the awareness that survivors may indeed experience problems and challenges after treatment. Listing all possible side effects according to diagnosis, stage, type of treatment, age, and comorbidities would fill volumes. Meanwhile, there is the recently identified need for guidelines, summaries, and plans to assist survivors through the challenging transition to life after cancer…a time when relief about the completion of treatments often collide with anxiety about recurrence and recovery.

Summaries, guidelines, and care plans

> *It is as if we have invented sophisticated techniques to save people from drowning, but once they have been pulled from the water, we leave them on the dock to cough and splutter on their own in the belief that we have done all that we can* [27].

Since the IOM *Lost in Transition* report identified the need for summaries, guidelines, and survivorship care plans, clinicians and researchers have been attempting to individualize follow-up care for cancer survivors [8,28,29]. According to this report, along with the follow-up report, *Implementing Survivorship Care Planning,* the general recommendation was made "that patients completing their primary treatment for cancer be given a summary of their treatment and a comprehensive plan for follow-up" [8,29]. (Table 3 lists specific components of a treatment summary.) This type of summary would include guidelines as a basis for the follow-up plan. The pediatric oncology community has guidelines demonstrated in the Children's Oncology Group Web site, *Cure Search* [30]. The book, *Survivors of Childhood Cancer: Assessment and Management*, has been available for oncology practitioners since 1994 [31]. Also, *Childhood Cancer Survivors: A Practical Guide to Your Future* has been available for the general public since 2000 and is considered the bible among younger cancer survivors and parents [32]. But adult oncology has lagged far behind in offering these

Table 3
Elements of survivorship care plan

Treatment summary	History of cancer treatment. Includes • Specific cancer diagnosis, including as many details as possible (stage, site, and date of diagnosis) • Treatments received, including type, dosages, dates, procedure, fields • Potential consequences, including problems encountered during treatment and their possible future impact
Follow-up plan	Future of cancer-related follow-up. Includes • Timing and content of recommended follow-up • Assessment and treatment of lingering effects • Examination and education regarding possible late effects • Recommended wellness plans (prevention practices, healthy behaviors, and screening) • Assessment for psychosocial distress and share information about resources locally and nationally • Evaluation for financial concerns (employment and insurance) with appropriate referrals

types of resources to their clients (Boxes 5 and 6 list Web sites that offer more survivorship resources).

Fortunately, the lack of information for survivors is changing in the adult oncology world. The ASCO has a committee to develop follow-up guidelines. ASCO decided to do this by systems rather than specific disease protocols. Cardiopulmonary guidelines were the first to be studied. After 2 years of work, a 40-page report was released, but no consensus for evidence-based guidelines was reached. It shows how difficult this task is in a population that has more than 100 different types of cancer, multiple stages of each disease, many therapies with different combinations and protocols, a wide range of ages, and comorbidities. The work will continue, however, and more reports will follow.

Although the NCCN develops disease-specific guidelines, it does not have much information in the way of long-term follow-up [33]. Hopefully, they soon will extend the type of excellent work they do with treatment decisions into extended guidelines for long-term survivors.

Meanwhile, one of the most exciting projects for survivorship follow-up is the Lance Armstrong Survivorship Center of Excellence Network that is currently funding multiple comprehensive cancer centers "to significantly

Box 5. General survivorship web sites

Many of these general sites link to more specific sites.
www.cancer.org—American Cancer Society
www.aicr.org—American Institute for Cancer Research
www.peoplelivingwithcancer.org—American Society of Clinical Oncology (ASCO)
www.acor.org—Association of Cancer Online Resources
www.cancercare.org—Cancer*Care*, Inc.
www.survivorshipguidelines.org—Children's Oncology Group
www.fertilehope.org—Fertile Hope
www.iom.edu—IOM
www.iccnetwork.org—Intercultural Cancer Council
www.livestrong.org—Livestrong/LAF
www.cancer.gov—NCI
www.canceradvocacy.org—NCCS
www.nccn.org—National Comprehensive Cancer Network (NCCN)
www.lymphnet.org—National Lymphedema Network
www.npaf.org—National Patient Advocate Foundation
www.cancerfatigue.org—Oncology Nursing Society site for fatigue
www.SurvivorsRetreat.com—Survivors' Retreat site

Box 6. Treatment summary templates

American Journal of Nursing Prescription for Living

The direct link to the printer-friendly template for the Prescription for Living Plan is available online at http://www.nursingcenter.com/library/static.asp?pageid=721732

The production of this template followed a series of meetings convened by the *AJN* and included key nursing organizations and leaders in 2006. *AJN* then published a special supplement that was dedicated entirely to survivorship issues. It also included articles and editorials around the Prescription for Living in the regular *AJN*.

American Society of Clinical Oncology: http://www.asco.org

ASCO has Cancer Treatment Summaries, Survivorship Care Plans, and Follow-up Care currently available for breast and colorectal cancers. The formats can be downloaded. Work continues on plans and follow-up care for different types of cancer.

Memorial Sloan Kettering Cancer Center

Offers an example of a one-page *Summary of Cancer Treatment and Follow-up Plan* that is being used and evaluated in their adult survivor clinics. The one-page format was requested by primary care providers (PCPs), and the template has online pull-down menus to increase usability. Can be viewed in *Implementing Cancer Survivorship Care Planning* [28].

Oncolink: Oncolife Survivorship Care Plan: www.oncolink.org/oncolife

From the Abramson Cancer Center of the University of Pennsylvania comes OncoLink, the Web's first cancer resource. This site is filled with all categories of resources, including a survivorship link to the OncoLife Survivorship Care Plan. Survivors can enter their treatment information and receive an individualized, basic care plan that can then be reviewed with their own health care team. It is meant to be a guide for a more in-depth discussion and personal interpretation with a physician or oncology provider.

Livestrong Survivorship Notebook from the Lance Armstrong Foundation

An organizational tool that helps organize information from the time of diagnosis through long-term survival. Sections include Cancer Survivor's Health Journal, Practical Information Summary, and Cancer Survivor's Medical Treatment Summary. Notebook can be ordered. Pages can be downloaded. http://www.livestrong.org/site/c.khLXK1PxHmF/b.2662947/k.9791/Get_Organized.htm

accelerate progress in the field of cancer survivorship" [34]. This hopefully will be accomplished through collaboration on joint projects that includes community partners as more survivors are seen in community settings than they are in academic centers. Oncology nurses are well represented on this project and are major contributors to model development and follow-up care.

More resources

Cancer Survivorship: Today and Tomorrow, edited by Patricia Ganz, MD, recently was published and includes extensive tables of physiologic and psychosocial morbidities and toxicities [35]. The IOM report, *Lost in Transition*, is a wealth of information about the delivery of survivorship care [8]. A new professional journal, the *Journal of Cancer Survivorship: Research and Practice*, delivered its first issue in March 2007 [36]. But for nurses, those in oncology and in all other areas of this diverse profession, there are recent publications dedicated to survivorship from a nursing perspective. Of particular interest is the 2006 *AJN* special supplement, *State of the Science Managing Late and Long-term Sequelae of Cancer and its Treatment* [23] along with companion articles in the April 2007 issue of *AJN*. Although the first publication focuses on the identification of survivorship issues that have an impact on the entire field of nursing in relation to survivorship, the second journal gives specific guidance in planning follow-up care for survivors. *The Cancer Survivor's Prescription for Living* offers a template to promote the routine survivorship care planning as recommended by the IOM report [37].

Although most of these journals are geared toward providers, there are publications directed toward consumers. *CURE: Cancer Updates, Research & Education* offers invaluable information and stories to patients undergoing cancer therapies, although its new companion, *Heal: Living Well After Cancer,* focuses on survivor or post-treatment issues [38,39]. Coping Magazine, MAMM, and Women & Cancer also offer support during therapy and beyond. All these resources hopefully will help providers and consumers to reduce the unknowns, smooth the transition from active treatment to life beyond cancer, and focus on how to be well with, through, and after cancer.

Models for follow-up

Survivors have needs that require a different model of care than what is currently available. One of the most controversial issues today is who is going to care for long-term cancer survivors and how. What type of follow-up is optimal; who will pay for this care and increased expense; and where will extra time and space be found to handle this expanding population? Also, will payers cover the expense of specialized follow-up without evidence-based guidelines? These questions are challenging not only for the oncology community but also for those in primary care as they attempt to create systems of care that have no track records. Meanwhile, another challenge is to find health care providers who have the experience, time, and desire to follow long-term survivors and can expedite referrals to appropriate specialists for timely diagnosis and treatment of potential problems.

Suggested models of follow-up care include

- Extension of care indefinitely from original clinic where oncologists continue to see their original patients indefinitely.
- Transition of care to nurse practitioner (NP), physician assistant, or PCP.
- Shared care with oncologist, NP, physician assistant, or PCP.
- Creation of survivorship subspecialty and clinic with dedicated staff and space.

The challenges are numerous and go beyond the basic question of who will fund these types of programs. Of paramount importance is who will be able to handle such increases in patient loads. Oncology clinics already are overloaded with more complicated patients who require longer periods of treatment. More oncologists will be retiring than are entering the field [40]. Primary care physicians are decreasing in numbers [41]. And the nursing shortage decreases the opportunities to educate more NPs. There are no easy answers to solving the problems within the current health care climate, but the first step surely is recognition of the needs, barriers, and challenges.

Final thoughts

Although oncology nurses focus on the delivery of care to newly diagnosed patients and those needing therapy, they rarely see long-term survivors after their initial follow-up. Oncology NPs sometimes have the responsibility to follow these survivors and monitor chronic or late effects, but these specialists are few and far between. But, as the authors state in *The Cancer Survivor's Prescription for Living,* "the management of symptoms related to cancer and cancer treatment falls within the scope of nursing practice, regardless of setting" [37]. The authors also describe nurses as catalysts, clinicians, educators, researchers, administrators, and advocates who are in excellent positions to provide effective, holistic, wellness-focused care, and care planning to survivors [42].

Although successes in treating cancer have dramatically increased the sheer numbers of survivors, these advancements have outpaced the availability to deliver adequate and responsible follow-up care. Multiple needs of cancer survivors, met and unmet, have been identified as have several barriers to the delivery of follow-up care. Meanwhile, resources are increasing. Models of care are being developed. Collaboration is replacing competition.

Survivors, along with their loved ones and health care providers, continue to work for better access to quality cancer care.

References

[1] Mullan F. Survivorship: a powerful place. In: Hoffman B, editor. A cancer survivor's almanac: charting your journey. Minneapolis (MN): Chronimed Publishing; 1996. p. XV–XIX.

[2] Sontag S. Illness as metaphor. New York: Random House; 1977.

[3] Leigh S. Myths, monsters and magic: personal perspectives and professional challenges of survival. Oncol Nurs Forum 1992;19:1475–80.

[4] Rowland J. Survivorship research: past, present, and future. In: Ganz P, editor. Cancer survivorship: today and tomorrow. New York: Springer; 2007. p. 28–42.

[5] Available at: http://seer.cancer.gov/csr/1975_2004/, based on November 2006 SEER data submission, posted to the SEER web site, 2007.

[6] Available at: http://cancercontrol.gov/ocs/prevalence/prevelence.html.

[7] Available at: http://www.cancer.org/docroot/STT/content/STT_1x_Cancer_Facts__Figures_2007.asp.

[8] Institute of Medicine. Hewitt M, Greenfield S, Stovall E, editors. From cancer patient to cancer survivor: lost in transition. Washington, DC: The National Academies Press; 2006. Available at: www.nap.edu.

[9] Leigh S. Cancer survivorship: a nursing perspective. In: Ganz P, editor. Cancer survivorship: today and tomorrow. New York: Springer; 2007. p. 8–13.

[10] Clark EJ, Stovall EL, Leigh S, et al. Imperatives for quality cancer care: access, advocacy, action & accountability. Silver Spring (MD): National Coalition for Cancer Survivorship; 1995.

[11] Available at: http://www.survivorship.cancer.gov.

[12] Available at: http://www.canceradvocacy.org.

[13] Institute of Medicine. Hewitt M, Weiner SL, Simone JV, editors. Childhood cancer survivorship: improving care and quality of life. Washington, DC: National Academies Press; 2003.

[14] Living beyond cancer: finding a new balance. President's cancer panel 2003 annual report. Bethesda (MD): U.S. Department of Health and Human Services, NIH, NCI; 2004.

[15] Centers for Disease Control, Lance Armstrong Foundation. A national action plan for cancer survivorship: advancing public health strategies. Atlanta (GA): U.S. Department of Health and Human Services, CDC; 2004.

[16] Institute of Medicine. Cancer care for the whole patient: meeting psychosocial health needs. Washington, DC: The National Academies Press; 2007. Prepublication copy released. Available at: www.nap.edu. Accessed October 23, 2007.

[17] Runowicz C, Haupt D. To be alive: a woman's guide to a full life after cancer. New York: Henry Holt & Company; 1995.

[18] Aziz N. Late effects of cancer treatment. In: Ganz P, editor. Survivorship: today and tomorrow. New York: Springer; 2007. p. 54–76.

[19] Ferrell BR, Hassey KH, Leigh S, et al. Quality of life in long-term cancer survivors. Oncol Nurs Forum 1995;22(6):915–22.

[20] The medical and psychological concerns of cancer survivors after treatment. In: Hewitt M, Greenfield S, Stovall E, editors. From cancer patient to cancer survivor: lost in transition. Washington, DC: The National Academies Press; 2006. p. 66–186.

[21] Leigh SA, Clark EJ. Psychosocial aspects of cancer survivorship. In: Berger AM, Portenoy RK, Weissman DE, editors. Principles and practice of supportive oncology. 2nd edition. Philadelphia: Lippincott-Raven Publishers; 2002. p. 1034–43.

[22] Grant M, Economou D, Ferrell B, et al. Preparing professional staff to care for cancer survivors. Journal of Cancer Survivorship: Research and Practice 2007;1(1):98–106.

[23] Curtiss CP, Haylock PJ, editors. State of the science on nursing approaches to managing late and long-term sequelae of cancer and cancer treatment, a special issue. Am J Nurs 2006;(Suppl).
[24] Pelusi J. Sexuality and body image. Am J Nurs 2006;(Suppl):32–8.
[25] Knobf MT. Reproductive and hormonal sequelae of chemotherapy in women. Am J Nurs 2006;(Suppl):60–5.
[26] Thaler-DeMers D. Endocrine and fertility effects in male cancer survivors. Am J Nurs 2006;(Suppl):66–71.
[27] Mullan F. Seasons of survival: reflections of a physician with cancer. N Engl J Med 1985;313: 270–3.
[28] American society of clinical oncology (ASCO). Available at: www.asco.org.
[29] Institute of Medicine. Implementing cancer survivorship care planning: workshop summary. Washington, DC: National Academies Press; 2007. Available at: www.nap.edu; www.iom.edu.
[30] Cure search at children's oncology group. Available at: www.survivorshipguidelines.org.
[31] Schwartz CL, Hobbie WL, Constine LS, et al. Survivors of childhood cancer: assessment and management. St. Louis (MO): Mosby; 1994.
[32] Keene N, Hobbie W, Ruccione K. Childhood cancer survivors: a practical guide to your future. Sebastopol (CA): O'Reilly; 2000.
[33] National comprehensive cancer network (NCCN). Available at: www.nccn.org.
[34] Available at: www.livestrong.org.
[35] Ganz P, editor. Cancer survivorship: today and tomorrow. New York: Springer; 2007.
[36] Journal of cancer survivorship: research and practice. New York: Springer.
[37] Haylock PJ, Mitchell SA, Cox T, et al. The cancer survivor's prescription for living. Am J Nurs 2007;107(4):58–70.
[38] CURE: cancer updates, research & education. Available at: www.curetoday.com.
[39] Heal: living well after cancer. Available at: www.healtoday.com.
[40] Erikson C, Salsberg E, Forte G, et al. Future supply and demand for oncologists: challenges to assuring access to oncology services. Journal of Oncology Practice 2007;3:79–86.
[41] Bodenheimer T. Primary care—will it survive? N Engl J Med 2006;355:861–4.
[42] Curtiss CP, Haylock PJ. Editorial: survivor-centered care. Am J Nurs 2006;(Suppl):4–5.

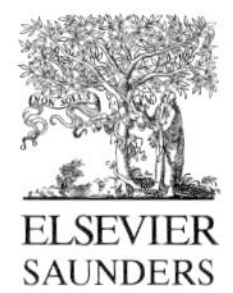

ELSEVIER
SAUNDERS

Nurs Clin N Am 43 (2008) 259–275

NURSING
CLINICS
OF NORTH AMERICA

Ethical Issues and Clinical Expertise at the End of Life

Karen J. Stanley, RN, MSN, AOCN, FAAN[a,*], Dawn Sawrun, MSN, APRN-BC, FNP, OCN[b], Marianne Treantafilos, MSN, APRN[b]

[a]*Pain and Palliative Care Service, Stamford Hospital, Stamford, CT, USA*
[b]*Nursing and Education, The Connecticut Hospice, Branford, CT, USA*

The landscape of oncology care has changed markedly in the past decade. Targeted therapies, the synergistic action of those therapies in combination with chemotherapy, intensity-modulated radiation therapy, advances in surgical precision (eg, video-assisted thoracic surgery), and second- and third-line therapies have extended the life span of patients who have cancer. These new therapies have created a patient population experienced in living with a life-threatening illness and a group that believes in the power of science and the ability of the health care system to find yet another therapy. It is especially difficult for patients, their families, and members of health care teams when the promise of new therapies has been exhausted and patients and families are faced with the expected yet unexpected.

These changes in the treatment paradigm have altered the nature of oncology nursing practice. Practitioners across the illness continuum are dealing with issues pertinent to end-of-life care for extended periods of time. These practitioners must consistently attend to physiologic and psychologic issues and balance the need for hope with the realities of current therapies. The integration of newer targeted therapies with their specific side-effect profiles that differ markedly from traditional chemotherapeutic agents and the sequelae to all types of cancer therapy also have changed care at the end of life. Strategies used to manage patients during the active treatment phase of illness can inform and improve nursing practice when active care has been set aside.

* Corresponding author. 111 Catalpa Road, Wilton, CT 06897.
E-mail address: kjstanley@optonline.net (K.J. Stanley).

doi:10.1016/j.cnur.2008.02.001

Nursing roles in palliative care have continued to expand. Clinical nurse specialists and nurse practitioners have joined their nursing colleagues in the multidisciplinary practice setting, having developed expertise in palliative care and symptom management that can be implemented along the illness continuum. Excellence in symptom management, an essential component of oncology care, has been supported by the Oncology Nursing Society in a strategic way. Putting Evidence Into Practice [1], an extensive and ongoing project, has defined and implemented an oncology nursing approach to evidence-based practice. Evidence-based practice is a process defined by (1) clinical questioning, (2) identifying best practice by critically appraising the evidence for validity and applicability, (3) actions of expert clinicians who apply the best evidence in light of patients' unique values and needs, and (4) evaluating the effectiveness of care and the continual improvement process [2]. In summary, evidence-based practice provides a guide to identify, critically appraise, and use evidence to solve clinical problems.

Cancer, aging, and comorbidities

During the next 20 years, the fastest-growing segment of the population will be the group aged 85 years and older, a reflection of positive trends in the management of chronic disease. The elderly have comorbid conditions that contribute an added symptom burden to the palliative care population. In the United States, 49% of noninstitutionalized individuals over 60 have two or more chronic conditions [3]. Individuals who have a history of multimodality and multiple cancer therapies can present with morbidities secondary to cancer therapy itself. These comorbidities and disabilities can present a challenge even for nurses skilled in symptom management and palliative care. Oncology nurses involved in active care can be proactive in providing clinical information about appropriate treatments and outcomes so that they might be integrated into the care plan across the continuum.

Selected ethical issues

Nursing's role on multidisciplinary teams has expanded to include more autonomous practice in managing symptoms under established standards of care. Expert nurses adjust medications and dosages, make multidisciplinary referrals, and engage patients at the most existential of levels as part of a normal day's work. This enlarged arena of nursing responsibility translates into greater ethical obligations. Distinguishing quality versus quantity of life, providing objective feedback about the patient's current status, articulating outcomes of health care decisions, and offering to be present as health care choices are clarified are activities that demonstrate nurses' commitment to these significant responsibilities.

The value of existence for its own sake, a false sense of security about technology and medicine's ability to rescue, and the need to maintain hope have obscured and postponed the inevitable need to confront critical issues. Ethical dilemmas on the micro and macro levels emerge daily as the debate on extending life versus postponing death continues. Today's demographic trends separate the generations and, as a consequence, many individuals and families have not lived with or cared for a dying person. A generation that has no practical or emotional experience with dying is bound to be uncomfortable with a multitude of issues surrounding end-of-life care.

Although cultural competency is essential across the illness continuum, nursing must be proactive in integrating cultural considerations into the palliative care arena. Race, ethnicity, gender, age, differing abilities, sexual orientation, religion, spirituality, and socioeconomic status [4] are reflected in patient and family values, norms, and customs. They shape how individuals make meaning out of illness, suffering, and death [5]. Perspectives on truth telling, decision making, withholding and withdrawing treatment, the experience of pain, symptom management, the meaning of food and nutrition, the meaning of a good death, and death rituals/mourning/practices are shaped by cultural beliefs [4]. Ensuring that understanding a particular culture's values, traditions, rites, and taboos holds true for particular patients and families prevents stereotypical responses. At the same time, nursing assessment should explore differences in values, needs, and concerns among patient and family members and ensure prioritization of patients' values.

Truth telling

Ethical principles are reflected not only in behavior but also in language [6]. Issues pertinent to all domains of care require communication such that goals and expectations can be articulated and those who are cared for can know and trust those providing the care. Over the continuum of care, oncology nurses often find themselves in circumstances that are ethically troublesome. Presenting truthful information to asked and unasked questions without destroying hope, providing information purposefully "filtered" because of patient or family wishes or cultural background, and confronting other members of a health team who obscure information are not uncommon.

Patient-focused communication requires prioritization of patients' interests. It is unethical to withhold information at the request of family members, friends, or other members of a health care team if a patient has expressed the desire to know and understand. When family members request a patient not be told the circumstances of the illness, these requests should be handled tactfully and respectfully by addressing the rationale for the request, the right of the patient to have the information, and an offer to be present during what others might see as a difficult and painful discussion.

If other members of a health care team request that a patient not be told, the nurse should explore the rationale for the request. If a practitioner evidences discomfort with the task of truth telling, nursing can speak to the ethical issues in this situation and offer to assist with the task. It is critical that members of health care teams are of one mind regarding truth telling and equally important they hold each other accountable for honoring this ethical commitment.

Delivering bad news is an essential part of practice in the palliative care arena. There is seldom disagreement in Western cultures that autonomous patients have the right to complete information regarding their illness, risks and benefits of interventions, and prognoses to make informed decisions. The ability to function as a patient advocate, however, is more complex than the verbalization of correct clinical data.

Truth telling occurs in the context of patients' wishes and emotional status. Confirming a patient's readiness to hear difficult news is an important first step. Reasonable ethical standards require that patients receive answers to difficult and frightening questions in a timely manner. Although this historically has been the physician's domain, the multidisciplinary structure of palliative care allows a modification of these role expectations in deference to a patient's best interest. The best possible case scenario is a rapid resolution of the unanswered questions by a member of the team who is able to answer correctly and empathetically and has the patient's confidence. Family members can be equally uncertain and anxious. With the patient's permission, they should be kept current as to the patient's status and expected outcomes.

If patients do not wish to be kept apprised of their health status and any changes that may occur, it is imperative to ask that a family member or friend be designated as a spokesperson and surrogate decision maker. In these instances it is appropriate to check in with patients periodically to ensure their initial instructions reflect their current thinking.

Withholding or withdrawing treatment

Withholding or withdrawing life-sustaining treatment is considered neither homicide nor suicide [7]. The courts have upheld the validity of Do Not Resuscitate and other treatment limitation orders, and there are no limits on the type of treatment that may be withheld or withdrawn. Withdrawal from a ventilator and withholding or withdrawing of parenteral nutrition and hydration may occur under the same conditions as any other medical treatment.

It is not unusual to withdraw modest treatments in an incremental way when the burdens outweigh the benefits. This is decided on an individual basis based on patients' wishes, if they can speak for themselves, or by designated family members or friends. Examples include discontinuing antihypertensive medications as blood pressure declines or reducing insulin dosage as appetite decreases. The underlying question that must be asked is, "Is this medication or intervention necessary at this time in the patient's life?"

In the majority of situations in which treatment or other interventions are providing no benefit, consensus is reached and life-sustaining interventions are not initiated or those underway may be stopped. It is at these moments that nursing can be particularly effective. Patients and families often require support for these difficult decisions, the repetition of medical data until a certain comfort level is reached, reconsideration of any potential therapies that might benefit patients, and, in some instances, permission to make the decision.

The decision to forgo further treatment moves patients and families into the final stage of the illness continuum and provides an opportunity for nursing to speak to what can be done. Reassurance about physical and psychologic comfort is always appropriate and essential for patients and their families. It also is important to query patients about any unstated fears (eg, respiratory distress, uncontrolled pain, or dying alone), so that a mutually agreed-on plan of care can be determined.

It is not unusual for patients or families to fear abandonment if they choose to forgo treatment. Abandonment can be subtle. Less time may be spent with patients and direct verbal engagement limited. Any of these behaviors may be viewed by the patients and families as emotional withdrawal at the least and abandonment at the worst [6]. Nursing can reassure patients and families that quality of life and comfort are now the primary goals and assist in decision making by reviewing options for sites of care and remaining emotionally available as decisions are made.

Requests for assistance in dying

Existential issues that confront oncology patients are no more evident than in discussions regarding assistance in dying. The adult patient's right to control health care interventions historically has allowed individuals to refuse to seek medical care, refuse or stop hydration and nutrition and other prescribed recommendations, and forgo or discontinue life support. These methods of ending life sooner have become commonplace. They are legally and morally acceptable to the majority of practitioners and have become a standard of practice for patients and health care teams [8].

It has been argued that withholding, withdrawing, or refusing treatment is no different, from a consequential perspective, from assistance in dying [9,10]. Others argue there is a distinct moral difference [11,12]. Although terminally ill residents of Oregon are able to receive prescriptions from their physicians for lethal medications that may be self-administered [13], all other jurisdictions in the United States have not legalized assistance in dying. The position of the Oncology Nursing Society on nurses' responsibility to patients requesting assistance in dying [14] recognizes that "individual nurses may encounter agonizing clinical situations and experience both personal and professional tension and ambiguity surrounding a patient's request for assistance in dying" [15]. It goes on to suggest that requests "should prompt a frank discussion of the rationale for the request, a thorough and nonjudgmental multidisciplinary assessment of the patient's unmet needs, and prompt and intensive intervention for previously unrecognized or unmet needs" [14].

For oncology nurses, the central issue is what can be done for patients who make this request. As suggested by the Oncology Nursing Society position [14], nurses should explore the reasons for the request, initiate a thorough multidisciplinary assessment of patients' needs, and ensure appropriate intervention. It may take considerable courage for a patient to initiate this discussion, and it is imperative that a professional, nonjudgmental response reflect a nurse's continued commitment to a patient's well-being. A nurse's moral conflict may reflect individual disapproval of the request, ambiguity regarding the "rightness" of the request, or a clear understanding that being sympathetic to the request does not allow compliance with the same.

What can nurses do? It is important to maintain eye contact and acknowledge the request, gently remind patients of the legal issues in that jurisdiction, explore the reason for the request, and discuss any unmet needs or concerns that need to be addressed. If there are fears about the future (eg, unmanaged symptoms), it is important to discuss how those symptoms will be managed effectively.

There never is a time when nothing more can be done, but there are times when a patient's request cannot be honored, a difficult position for patients and care providers. Honesty, integrity, evidence-based care, concern for patients and families, and specific attendance to the problems at hand are important nursing interventions.

Expert management of clinical issues

Meaningful conversations cannot occur in the midst of unrelieved symptoms. Nurses must advocate for and contribute to effective symptom management. Expert practice, holding others accountable for that same standard of excellence, and continually advocating for patients until symptoms are well controlled are essential practice components [16]. These unmanaged symptoms can strip patients of their dignity, impose tremendous professional and ethical burdens on nurses, and destroy the quality of life of patients and families [17]. The selected symptoms are those that are most difficult to manage at the end of life and cause anguish for all involved. It is ironic that in some instances the expert management of symptoms can bring its own ethical dilemmas. In most instances, the underlying cause of the symptom cannot be "fixed," and the symptom itself may be only palliated. In those instances (eg, delirium, terminal restlessness, and intractable pain), when expert clinical intervention does not palliate the symptom effectively, sedation may be used to minimize patient anguish, physical and psychologic.

Bleeding

End-stage bleeding needs to be evaluated thoroughly before a treatment decision is made. Potential causes include thrombocytopenia, HIV, hepatic disease, tumor progression with eroding vessels, hemorrhagic masses, and friable tissues. Treatment considerations include the amount of bleeding present, patient level of awareness, and patient comfort level.

Treatments available for consideration are topical thrombin, Gelfoam, and silver nitrate to help control small amounts of localized bleeding. Waller and Caroline [18] recommend the use of gauze soaked in 1:1000 epinephrine over the bleeding point or application of sucralfate paste over widespread oozing. It is more difficult to manage those patients at risk for extensive and life-threatening bleeding. For those whose bleeding cannot be controlled successfully, use of a benzodiazepine in doses adequate to sedate patients can ease fears and minimize awareness of the circumstances. Bleeding is visually difficult and the use of red towels to absorb bleeding can ease the anguish for families who want to remain close to a patient. It is impossible, however, to completely disguise and disregard. Patients and families should be reassured that it will be handled as sensitively and effectively as possible and that the goal of care continues to be maximization of quality of life.

Dyspnea

Dyspnea, or the uncomfortable awareness of breathing, is a common symptom at the end of life affecting up to 75% of this population [19,20]. Patients who have respiratory disease fear this symptom above all. Causes include primary or metastatic lung disease, pleural effusion, pulmonary fibrosis, and airway obstruction from progressive tumor growth. Chronic obstructive pulmonary disease, congestive heart failure (CHF), asthma, pneumonia, anemia, anxiety, pulmonary embolism and cachexia can exacerbate the problem [21–23]. Dyspnea is a subjective experience and can be affected by psychologic factors. Anxiety can exacerbate dyspnea, which in turn is affected by the anxiety.

In the palliative care setting, extensive workups generally do not occur; the focus shifts to assessing and managing the primary symptom and any associated symptoms, such as anxiety. When it is not possible to treat the underlying disease successfully, symptom management is paramount. Treatment considerations likely center on the cause of the dyspnea. For example, if a patient has dsypnea associated with CHF, it might be treated most effectively with a diuretic.

The most common pharmacologic intervention for dyspnea at the end of life is an opioid analgesic, typically morphine, although other opioids are used successfully [22,24]. Opioid analgesics function by reducing oxygen demand and dilating pulmonary vessels, which in turn reduce preload to the heart [21]. In studies of patients who had cancer, morphine did not compromise respiratory function as measured by respiratory effort, oxygen saturation, or respiratory rate [25]. Twycross [26] has suggested that early intervention with morphine or another opioid might prolong survival by reducing physical and psychologic distress and exhaustion.

Other possible interventions include bronchodilators, corticosteroids, sedatives, and tranquilizers. Bronchodilators help open up the airways; corticosteroids help decease inflammation and mucous production [22]; and benzodiazepines reduce anxiety and, therefore, decrease oxygen demand [24]. Regardless of the cause, severe dyspnea is an emergency and should be treated aggressively. The combination of an opioid and sedative can markedly relieve patients who have end-stage disease [27].

Terminal congestion

Terminal congestion, or "death rattle," commonly occurs in up to 92% of patients in the hours immediately before death, most commonly when there is a decreased level of consciousness [20,28]. The audible sound of congestion that is heard is air passing over or through pooled secretions in the oropharnyx or bronchi [20]. Although this is not believed to be painful for patients, it often is a source of distress for families, friends, and caregivers.

Possible causes include inhibition of normal secretion clearance, inability to swallow, decreased cough reflex, a supine recumbent position, or possible dysfunction of the cilia that help move secretions up to be cleared [20,28]. Comorbid conditions include infection, chronic obstructive pulmonary disease, CHF, pulmonary embolism, and dysphasia [20].

Assessment should focus on treatable underlying causes when appropriate and according to the wishes of patients and families. For example, pneumonia could be treated with antibiotics or CHF/fluid overload with a diuretic. When this is not possible, anticholinergic medications, such as glycopyrrolate (Robinul), atropine sulfate, and hyoscine hydrobromide (scopolamine), are the treatments of choice [20]. These medications help reduce the amount of bronchial secretions produced. Although glycopyrrolate has the advantage of producing less sedation and agitation, hyoscine hydrobromide is more effective and is the medication used most widely for the treatment of terminal congestion when patient alertness is less a priority [28]. In an open-label study, 56% of patients receiving hyoscine hydrobromide had a significantly reduced noise level after 30 minutes compared with 27% of patients who had received glycopyrrolate [29].

The most effective nonpharmacologic treatment is positioning in a semiprone position, which promotes postural drainage of these pooled secretions [28]. Suctioning usually is not recommended, because it can be uncomfortable and cause significant agitation and distress.

Teaching patients and families is critically important when managing this distressing symptom. The term, "death rattle," should be avoided and "respiratory congestion" substituted. Nurses can explain that it is a common symptom at the end of life, the reasons for its occurrence, and recommended interventions. If patients are cared for at home, families should be instructed in relieving the symptom.

Wound care

Wound care is an important palliative care issue as untreated wounds can lead to physical discomfort and impair quality of life. The focus of wound care in palliative settings is the management of related symptoms, such as odor, exudate, bleeding, pain, and infection.

Patients at the end of life are at risk for skin breakdown because of fragile skin, excess pressure and friction, lack of proper nutrition, compromised mobility, dehydration, incontinence, advanced age, surgical wounds, fistulas, stomas, fungating tumors, peripheral edema, and lymphedema [23,30,31]. Often as death approaches the skin begins to fail because of increased pressure and altered perfusion, which put patients at risk for further breakdown. It is important to inform patients and families that the wounds have limited chance of healing. When this is true, it is of primary importance to ascertain the goals of patients and their families [32] (eg, pain control with fewer dressing changes versus odor control with more frequent dressing changes).

Topical anesthetics can be used in the wound bed to manage lower levels of pain [32]. Pain that is moderate to severe should be managed pharmacologically. Crushed metronidazole also can be sprinkled into the wound bed to help decrease odor and the amount of exudate from the wound [32]. Dressings should be selected carefully with the intention of minimizing trauma with dressing changes and preventing further deterioration of the wound or surrounding skin [31]. Skin barriers should be used for at-risk areas rather than adhesive dressings as this helps to preserve the integrity of the fragile skin [31]. As is true with many other symptoms at the end of life, it is difficult to acknowledge what cannot be "healed." In any conversation with patients and families, the emphasis should be on what can be done.

Delirium and terminal restlessness

In 1997, an Australian nurse deemed terminal restlessness "a palliative care emergency" [33]. Although only one of myriad symptoms experienced at the end of life, delirium may be the most distressing to patients and families. It forces a premature separation of patients and loved ones, leaves unfinished business and unspoken words, and, often, caregivers in conflict in the absence of advance directives. It has been identified as the third most common reason for inpatient admission of terminally ill hospice patients [34] and in a national survey of hospice nurses considered the most difficult symptom to manage at the end of life [35]. Lawlor and Bruera [36] describe delirium as a "transient global disorder of cognition and attention." The idea that it can be transient is significant, as early detection and intervention can improve quality of life and reduce anguish for the patients and caregivers/families even if for a brief interval before death.

Risk factors for the development of delirium include advanced age, prior cognitive impairment, illness severity, and comorbid factors. There are many potential causes, including environmental factors, metabolic or endocrine disorders, infection, nutritional deficits, central nervous system malignancy, seizures, hypoxia, withdrawal from alcohol or prescribed or illicit drugs, fluid imbalance, and medications commonly used at the end of life (eg, opioids, corticosteroids, tricyclic antidepressants, benzodiazepines, nonsteroidal anti-inflammatory drugs, H_2-blockers, and scopolamine) [37].

The cardinal signs of delirium are acute onset; a change in cognition that cannot be explained by a pre-existing or evolving conditions; reduced ability to focus, sustain, or shift attention; and physiologic data that may account for the disturbance [37]. A common feature is disinhibition, in which emotions normally under control are exaggerated [21]. Patients repeatedly and irrationally may make demands to be taken home or may cry out uncontrollably when approached or touched. This may be misinterpreted as pain or escalating delirium and lead to the destructive triangle, a response to misinterpreted cues that results in administration of more opioids or the addition of benzodiazepines or other medications that actually exacerbate the delirium [36].

Correction and treatment of underlying disorders are complex issues in the hospice and palliative population. Each case must be considered within an individual context of the philosophy and goals of hospice and palliative care, patient and family goals and expectations, the life expectancy of patients, and the benefit versus burden on or risk for patients.

Research supports the use and safety of hydration to attempt reversal of delirium when the suspected cause is toxicity related to the M3G and M6G metabolites of morphine [38]. Morphine dose reduction and opioid rotation are interventions that can be used concomitantly with hydration to reverse the M3G and M6G toxicity.

Haloperidol frequently is named as a first-line pharmacologic intervention for the management of delirium whereas chlorpromazine is cited as a second-line medication, possibly as effective as haloperidol, although both may cause extrapyramidal side effects if given over a long period of time. Both seem to improve cognitive function. The addition of lorazepam is suggested when extrapyramidal side effects, myoclonus or twitching, are present, or when rapid or deeper sedation is needed [36–40]. The newer atypical antipsychotic medications, olanzapine and risperidone, offer a better side-effect profile, having no anticholinergic or extrapyramidal effects, but come with these caveats: they were formulated for geriatric populations and may have no benefit for the terminally ill; they are costly; they have not been studied systematically for the treatment of delirium; and recent reports have warned of a possible increased risk for stroke [37]. Phenobarbital, lorazepam, and midazolam are used when much deeper sedation is required, as in cases of terminal restlessness that do not respond to the aforementioned medications [37,40–42].

Dosing and routes for quelling delirium and terminal restlessness depend on the severity of the agitation, the level of cognitive impairment, the level of arousal, and the ability of patients to swallow. Parenteral administration frequently is required, and although many treatment algorithms can be found in the literature, patient assessment and clinical judgment always guide treatment options. Table 1 lists recommendations for the pharmacologic management of delirium and terminal restlessness.

Palliative sedation

Despite the most rigorous attempts to control symptoms at the end of life, many patients develop intractable or refractory symptoms. A retrospective study by Kohara and colleagues [44] revealed that 54% of patients had more than one refractory symptom at the end of life. One has only to witness the dyspnea of end-stage cardiac or pulmonary disease or the persistent emesis of patients who have bowel obstruction to understand the anguish of patients and families when the best efforts of expert clinicians do not bring expected and often promised relief. Terminal restlessness and rapidly escalating pain also bring patients, caregivers, and professionals to the brink of despair.

A standard palliative treatment to relieve the physical distress of these symptoms, referred to as palliative sedation, often is initiated at the very end of life and based on a set of guiding principles and procedures. The use of palliative sedation remains controversial, misunderstood, and somewhat contentious. To guide patients and their caregivers through the complex and emotionally fraught issues involved in the initiation of palliative sedation, nurses must understand the ethical, legal, and moral implications and have the expertise to administer, monitor, and properly document the course of palliative sedation. As in all aspects of end-of-life care, palliative sedation requires an exploration of personal values and beliefs, acceptance, and understanding of an institution's practice protocols and a supportive and trusting interdisciplinary team.

The Hospice and Palliative Nurses Association defines palliative sedation as "the monitored use of medication intended to induce varying degrees of unconsciousness, but not death, for relief of refractory and unendurable symptoms in imminently dying patients" [45]. Cherney and Portenoy [46] defined refractory symptoms as those that did not respond to aggressive trials of the usual treatments over a reasonable period of time and were unlikely to be adequately controlled by more invasive or noninvasive therapies without excessive or intolerable side effects or complications.

Table 1
Pharmacologic therapy for delirium and terminal restlessness: general guidelines

Haloperidol: oral	0.5–5 mg every 8 hours [43]
	2 mg orally or subcutaneously every 6 hours and 2 mg every 1 hour as needed for severe agitation. Reduce dose when effect achieved; if not, move to chlorpromazine with palliative consult [21].
	Up to 20 mg for 24 hours usually sufficient for the elderly starting with 0.5–1 mg orally every hour until effect achieved; then reduce to 1–3 mg for 24 hours with as-needed doses available [37].
Haloperidol: subcutaneous, intramuscular, or intravenous	0.5–2 mg per titrating dose to clinical effect hourly intravenously; 0.2–1 mg per hour maintenance—EKG monitoring recommended to observe for prolonged QTC with intravenous infusion [43].
	0.5–1 mg subcutaneously twice a day if mild; if severe, 0.5–1 mg every hour until under control, then reduce dose to every 6–8 hours [40].
	Up to 20 mg per 24 hours usually sufficient for the elderly starting with 0.5–1 mg every hour until effect achieved; then reduce to 1–3 mg per 24 hours with as-needed doses available: parenteral doses are approximately twice as strong as oral doses [37].
Chlorpromazine: oral, intramuscular, or intravenous	12.5–50 mg every 8–12 hours. Sedative, anticholinergic, and hypotensive effects [43].
	If patient is refractory and life expectancy measured in days (terminal restlessness), chlorpromazine ± lorazepam [40].
	May use as alternative to haloperidol (no dose recommendation) [37].
Risperidone: oral	From 0.5 mg per day to 2–4 mg per day. In the elderly has less extrapyramidal effect [16].
	May use as alternative to haloperidol at 0.5–1 mg orally twice a day [17].
	May use as alternative to haloperidol 0.5–1 mg orally twice a day [7].
Olanzapine: oral	5 mg at bedtime, titrated to effect [43].
	May use as alternative to haloperidol at 2.5–15 mg orally per 24 hours [40].
	May use as alternative to haloperidol at 2.5–20 mg per 24 hours in divided doses [37].
Quetiapine: oral or sublingual	May use as alternative to haloperidol at 50–100 mg orally twice a day [40].
Lorazepam: oral, sublingual, subcutaneous, or intravenous	0.5–2 mg every 4–8 hours if anxiolytic effects required or if myoclonus present [43].
	Add lorazepam for refractory agitation despite high doses of neuroleptics at 0.5–2 mg every 4–6 hours sublingually or intravenously [40].
	Add to haloperidol when rapid sedation needed; do not use as single agent [37].
Midazolam: subcutaneous or intravenous	20–100 mg per 24 hours continuous infusion for sedation in refractory cases. 3–5 mg priming dose if rapid sedation required. Start infusion with 1 mg per hour; dose should be titrated frequently to effect [43]
	30–100 mg subcutaneously per 24 hours continuous infusion for sedation in refractory cases [37].

Data from Refs [21,37,40,43].

Palliative sedation may vary in duration of therapy and depth of sedation. Titration based on the needs of patients is an achievable goal and sometimes can be patient directed. Temporary sedation for 24 to 48 hours may be trialed to break the symptom cycle and obviate deep sedation.

Deep, uninterrupted sedation until a patient dies, however, frequently is required to provide relief from refractory symptoms.

In Vacco v. Quill [47], the United States Supreme Court ruled against euthanasia but supported the use of palliative sedation when used to relieve refractory symptoms. Controversy continues over what comprises a refractory symptom and whether or not palliative sedation should be used for physical suffering only or applied in situations of spiritual or existential suffering. Part of the dilemma rests in that there is no objective scale to measure this kind of suffering, and some refer to the slippery slope of assisting patients to die rather that palliating symptoms. Some hospice practitioners believe strongly in the possibility of transcendence by working through spiritual issues at the end of life and thus eschew palliative sedation. However, patient autonomy should dictate the treatment, and practitioners theoretically opposed are obligated to relinquish care to unbiased providers.

Based on the principles of autonomy and beneficence, the doctrine of double effect has four basic tenets that guide practitioners in the ethical justification of palliative sedation. The doctrine of double effect facilitates an understanding of intent and clarifies the lines between assistance in dying, euthanasia, and sedation for refractory distress. The doctrine of double effect states that an action with two possible effects is permitted if the action is not in itself immoral, is undertaken only with the intent of achieving the possible good effect, does not bring about the possible good effect by means of the possible bad effect (ie, death is not the means to relieve the suffering), and is undertaken for a proportionately grave reason (ie, the urgency of a patient's need for relief).

The Hospice and Palliative Nurses Association summarizes this principle simply by stating that although death is foreseen, palliative sedation is intended to relieve suffering [45].

In Brajtman's qualitative research [48] on the experiences of hospice professionals and families witnessing patients who have terminal restlessness, several themes emerged:

1. Families cannot bear to witness unrelieved suffering and ask for intervention. Sedation of patients helps staff cope with the stress of family suffering.
2. Administering medication helps maintain control and increases confidence in handling the crises of patients and families when suffering occurs. Negotiating with families over increasing or decreasing dosing restores control, helping family members feel that the team is accepting and empathetic.
3. Ambivalence exists in caregivers and team members over the use of strong sedatives, and the degree of suffering often is assessed differently by family members and members of health care teams. There is not always full agreement among a health care team regarding the degree of suffering or the level of sedation that is needed.

Brajtman's work highlights the importance of family education and the ability of staff to read family and patient cues and to deliver information such that it can be received. It underscores the utmost importance of palliating symptoms to the fullest extent and in including all team members and family members or caregivers in discussions when palliative sedation is presented as a last resort intervention.

There is consensus in the literature regarding the need for an organized and thoughtful approach to palliative sedation. Four conditions must be present before palliative sedation is considered: a terminal diagnosis; symptoms that are refractory and cause extreme distress; a signed, active Do Not Resuscitate order; and death expected within hours to days.

Prognostication has remained a challenge, but several scales, such as the Palliative Performance Scale [41], can guide practitioners when considering the implementation of palliative sedation. Care must be taken that all refractory symptoms are assessed and aggressive interventions attempted by palliative care practitioners, an expanding role for advanced practice nurses (APNs). Rousseau [42] suggests ethical, psychiatric, or spiritual consultation as needed, including family counseling, to resolve family discord if present.

Once the four conditions are established, protocols must be in place to assure autonomy, informed consent, technical expertise, and ongoing interdisciplinary and family/caregiver communication, the very themes uncovered by Brajtman's research. Nurses function as patient advocates and expert clinicians and must have the necessary communication skills to initiate discussions of palliative sedation. In the best scenario, patients have clarified their wishes regarding sedation versus consciousness at the time of admission to hospice. When patients' wishes for sedation versus intractable suffering are documented at admission, the burden on family members to make difficult decisions and often the ambivalence felt among team members can be mitigated.

This scenario can be instructive in significant ways. When querying patients about their wishes regarding palliative or hospice care, an interdisciplinary team can clarify what patients would wish done if circumstances were such that palliative sedation were a reasonable option. It is more important to have this conversation when it can be reasonably predicted that patients would need palliative sedation in the days or weeks ahead. APNs are well trained to educate bedside caregivers, including families, regarding cues that signal a need to titrate medication for sedative purposes or to prevent breakthrough symptoms of a previously present symptom, such as pain or myoclonus. APNs also can develop policies and procedures to educate staff about documentation requirements regarding patients' and families' responses to palliative sedation and can assist in keeping communication open, clear, and consistent among family and team members [41,42].

Midazolam frequently is cited as effective for palliative sedation along with other benzodiazepines and barbiturates. Chlorpromazine, haloperidol, and propofol also are used [37,41,42]. Midazolam is favored because it is fast acting, has a short half-life, can be given continuously via subcutaneous infusion, and is easily titrated [37]. Midazolam can be initiated at 0.5 to 1 mg per hour subcutaneously or intravenously or, if more rapid sedation is needed, a bolus dose of 3 to 5 mg may be given. The infusion then may be titrated from its starting point by 1 mg per hour to a maintenance dosage of 20 to 120 mg per day [37,42]. Table 1 lists medications and doses suggested by palliative experts in the management of delirium and terminal restlessness, essentially the same medications used for palliative sedation.

Before initiating palliative sedation, it is important to fully discuss with families which interventions and medications will be continued and which discontinued. All medications previously used to control symptoms, such as anticonvulsants for seizures, scopolamine for secretions, and opioids for pain, should continue, although doses usually are not advanced unless there is a clear need for titration. Interventions, such as total parental nutrition or other forms of nutrition and hydration, are complex issues, and discussions with families or caregivers may best be held with interdisciplinary team members present, such as pastoral care or social work. As patients under palliative sedation begin to die, some families may express ambivalence and helplessness. Nurses at the bedside can provide ongoing reinforcement of families' decisions and continuing education and support, alleviating anxiety through compassionate and knowledgeable care.

Although the practice of palliative sedation remains controversial even within the hospice and palliative professional communities, nurses engaged in end-of-life care need to look deep within themselves to examine their own belief systems, reconcile their beliefs with the ethical underpinnings of this humanistic intervention, and find the courage to advocate for dying patients. Nursing, steeped in the traditions of caring, empathy, and communication and providing evidence-based practice, also can provide support to all team members, the kind of support that maintains the cohesiveness of a well-functioning team. It is incumbent on hospice and palliative nurses to recognize untreated refractory symptoms and to speak with confidence predicated on a sound knowledge base and ethical principles. The final goal always is death with dignity for all patients.

References

[1] Gobel BH, Beck SL, O'Leary C. Nursing-sensitive patient outcomes: the development of the putting evidence into practice resources for nursing practice. Clin J Oncol Nurs 2006;10(5): 621–4.

[2] DePalma J. Evidence-based clinical practice guidelines. Semin Perioper Nurs 2000;9(3): 115–20.

[3] Foley D, Brock D. Demography and epidemiology of dying in the U.S. with emphasis on deaths of older persons. Hosp J 1998;13:49–60.

[4] Mazanec P, Panke JT. Cultural considerations in palliative care. In: Ferrell BR, Coyle N, editors. Textbook of palliative nursing. 2nd edition. New York: Oxford University Press; 2006.

[5] Kagawa-Singer M, Blackhall L. Negotiating cross-cultural issues at the end of life. JAMA 2001;286:2993–3001.

[6] Stanley KJ. The healing power of presence: respite from the fear of abandonment. Oncol Nurs Forum 2002;29:935–40.

[7] Barber v. Superior Court 147CalAppd 1006, 195 Cal Rptr 484. (CalCt App, 2nd Dist 1983).

[8] Quill TE, Lee BC, Nunn S. Palliative treatments of last resort: choosing the least harmful alternative. University of Pennsylvania Center for Bioethics Assisted Suicide Consensus Panel. Arch Intern Med 2000;132:488–93.

[9] Schwarz JK. Understanding and responding to patients' requests for assistance in dying. J Nurs Scholarsh 2003;35:377–84.

[10] Quill TE, LB, Brock DW. Palliative options of last resort: a comparison of voluntarily stopping eating and drinking, terminal sedation, physician-assisted suicide, and voluntary active euthanasia. JAMA 1997;278:2099–104.

[11] Pellegrino ED. Compassion needs reason too. JAMA 1993;270:874–5.

[12] Bleich JD. Life as an intrinsic rather than instrumental good: the "spiritual" case against euthanasia. Issues Law Med 1993;9:139–49.

[13] Oregon Death with Dignity Act. 1997. Oregon Revised Statute 127800-127: 897.

[14] Oncology Nursing Society. The nurse's responsibility to the patient requesting assistance in dying. Available at: http://www.ons.org/publications/positions/AssistedSuicide.shtml. Accessed September 7, 2007.

[15] Volker DL. Oncology nurses' experiences with requests for assisted dying from terminally ill patients with cancer. Oncol Nurs Forum 2001;28:39–49.

[16] American Nurses Association. Position statement: pain management and control of distressing symptoms in dying patients. Available at: http://www.nursingworld.org/MainMenuCategories/HealthcareandPolicyIssues/ANAPositionStatements/EthicsandHumanRights/etpain14426.aspx. Accessed November 2, 2007.

[17] Brant JM. The art of palliative care: living with hope, dying with dignity. Oncol Nurs Forum 1998;25:995–1004.

[18] Waller A, Caroline NL. Smelly tumors. In: Waller A, Caroline NL, editors. Handbook of palliative care in cancer. Boston: Butterworth-Heinemann; 1996.

[19] LaDuke S. Terminal dyspnea and palliative care: patient deaths are inevitable. 'Bad deaths'—those accompanied by severe suffering—are not. Am J Nurs 2001;101(11):26–31.

[20] Dudgeon D. Dyspnea, death rattle, and cough. In: Ferrell BR, Coyle N, editors. Textbook of palliative nursing. 2nd edition. New York: Oxford University Press; 2006.

[21] Reddy S, Elsayem A, Talukdar R. Pain management and symptom control. In: Kantarjian H, Wolff RA, Koller CA, editors. MD Anderson manual of medical oncology. New York: McGraw-Hill; 2006.

[22] Kvale P, Simoff M, Prakash U. Palliative care. Chest 2003;123(1):284–311.

[23] Pappagallo M, Dickerson E, Varga J, et al. Pain. Heidrich D. Skin lesions. Spencer P. Dyspnea. In: Kuebler K, Esper P, editors. Palliative practices A–Z for the bedside clinician. Pittsburgh: Oncology Nursing Society; 2002.

[24] LeGrand S. Dyspnea: the continuing challenge of palliative management. Curr Opin Oncol 2002;14(4):394–8.

[25] Bruera E, Macmillan K, Pither J, et al. Effects of morphine on the dyspnea of terminal cancer patients. J Pain Symptom Manage 1990;5(6):341–4.

[26] Twycross R. Morphine and dyspnoea. In: Twycross R, editor. Pain relief in advanced cancer. New York: Churchill Livingstone; 1994.

[27] Ventafridda V, Spoldi E, De Conno F. Control of dyspnea in advanced cancer patients. Chest 1990;981:1544–5.

[28] Owens D. Management of upper airway secretions at the end of life. J Hospice Palliat Nurs 2006;8(1):12–4.

[29] Back IN, Jenkins K, Blower A, et al. A study comparing hyoscine hydrobromide and glycopyrrolate in the treatment of death rattle. Palliat Med 2001;15:329–36.

[30] Richards A, Kelechi T, Hennessy W. Risk factors and wound management for palliative care patients. J Hospice Palliat Nurs 2007;9(4):179–81.

[31] Hughes R, Bakos A, O'Mara A, et al. Palliative wound care at the end of life. Home Health Care Management Practice 2005;17(3):196–202.

[32] Tice M. Wound care in the face of life-limiting illness. Home Healthc Nurse 2006;24(2): 115–8.

[33] Burke AL. Palliative care: an update on 'terminal restlessness'. Med J Aust 1997;166(1): 1042–54.

[34] Head B, Faul A. Terminal restlessness as perceived by hospice professionals. Amer J Hosp Palliat Med 2005;22:277–82.

[35] Johnson DC, Kassner J, Houser J, et al. Barriers to effective symptom management in hospice. J Pain Symptom Manage 2004;29(1):69–79.

[36] Lawler PG, Bruera E. Delirium in patients with advanced cancer. Hematol Oncol Clin North Am 2002;16(3):701–14.

[37] Breitbart W, Strout C. Delirium in the terminally ill. Clin Geriatr Med 2000;16(2):357–69.

[38] Casarett DJ, Inouye SK. Diagnosis of delirium near the end of life. Ann Intern Med 2001; 135(1):32–40.

[39] Bruera E, Sala R, Rico MA, et al. Effects of parenteral hydration in terminally ill cancer patients: a preliminary study. J Clin Oncol 2005;23(10):2366–71.

[40] National Comprehensive Cancer Network. Clinical practice guidelines in oncology. Palliative care. V.1.2006.

[41] Sinclair CT, Stephenson RC. Palliative sedation: assessment, management, and ethics. Hosp Physician Mar 2006;33–8.

[42] Rosseau P. Palliative sedation in the management of refractory symptoms. J Support Oncol 2004;2(2):181–6.

[43] Caraceni A, Martini C, Simonetti F. Neurological problems in advanced cancer. In: Doyle D, Hanks G, Cherny N, et al, editors. Oxford textbook of palliative medicine. 3rd edition. New York: Oxford University Press; 2005.

[44] Kohara J, Eoka H, Takayama H, et al. Sedation in terminally ill patients with cancer with uncontrollable physical distress. J Palliat Med 2005;8:20–5.

[45] Hospice and Palliative Nurses Association. Palliative sedation at the end of life. Available at: http://www.hpna.org/pdf/PositionStatement_PalliativeSedation.pdf.

[46] Cherney NI, Portenoy RK. Sedation in the management of refractory symptoms: guidelines for evaluation and treatment. J Palliat Care 1994;11(2):31–8.

[47] Vacco v. Quill, 117 Sct 2293 (1997).

[48] Brajtman S. Helping the family through the experience of terminal restlessness. J Hosp Palliat Nurs 2005;7:73–81.

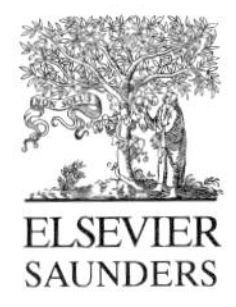

ELSEVIER
SAUNDERS

Nurs Clin N Am 43 (2008) 277–282

NURSING
CLINICS
OF NORTH AMERICA

War on Cancer: Victory or Defeat?

Joyce P. Griffin-Sobel, PhD, RN, AOCN, APRN-BC, CNE

Hunter-Bellevue School of Nursing, Hunter College, 425 East 25th Street, Suite 503, New York, NY 10010, USA

In 1971, then President Richard Nixon launched the "War on Cancer" by signing the National Cancer Act and proposing "an intensive campaign to find a cure for cancer," although he never used the word "war." The Cancer Act was driven by the actions of New York philanthropist, Mary Lasker, who mobilized political and public support for its passage over the protests of the medical establishment [1].

It is comforting to health professionals in oncology to proclaim that the War on Cancer has been won. Is that an accurate description, however, of the current state of affairs in cancer care? A recent editorial in the *Wall Street Journal*, written by an oncologist, criticized the National Cancer Institute, the Centers for Disease Control and Prevention, and the American Cancer Society for hailing a 2% decline in cancer mortality rates [2]. He cites these gaps in cancer care as examples: poor colonoscopy screening rates, often because physicians forget to recommend the procedure; poor colonoscopy technique by less-skilled operators, resulting in lower detection of polyps; prostate cancer surgeries performed by inexperienced physicians, resulting in less than optimal cancer control; and patients unable to obtain the pain medications prescribed by their oncologists because pharmacies have inadequate supplies. Health care access disparities and gaps in care, particularly in lower socioeconomic areas, are well documented, so it is difficult to support the contention of a victory over cancer for many Americans.

Victories

Although a review of medical oncology therapy advances is beyond the scope of this article, dramatic advances have been made in treatment of many cancers. Targeted therapies have created a paradigm shift in cancer

E-mail address: jgri@hunter.cuny.edu

0029-6465/08/$ - see front matter
doi:10.1016/j.cnur.2008.02.005

treatment by directly interfering with the malignant growth process. As part of the Human Genome Project, investigators in the Cancer Genetics Branch have made significant advances in determining the genetic contribution to cancer development and progression. The identification of inherited mutations involved in some cancers has led to significant therapeutic advances. Patients who have breast, colorectal, and lung cancer currently benefit directly from these advances.

How would a victory over cancer be defined? This writer suggests a victory would include equal access for all to quality cancer care, including effective and timely preventive and screening care, and expert clinical care by health care practitioners. Some success has been made in reducing cancer risk factors. Tobacco use in the United States has declined; although the prevalence of smoking in adults remained stable between the years of 1990 and 2004, the number of cigarettes smoked per day decreased [3]. The use of hormone therapy in women has substantially decreased since the 2002 publication of the Women's Health Initiative trial, which demonstrated a higher risk for breast cancer and cardiovascular disease with its use. Breast cancer incidence has declined significantly since 1999 as a result of mammography screening and a decline in the use of hormone therapy [3].

Significant advances have been made in nursing research. Several nurse researchers have contributed to the bodies of work in the areas of fatigue, symptom distress, cancer survivorship issues, sexuality and body image, sleep disturbances, psychosocial states and coping, quality of life, family systems changes, and so forth. Tobacco cessation strategies have been the subject of research studies done by nurses. The amount of nursing research, however, leaves much room for improvement. A systematic review of oncology nursing research [4] shows that the five most frequently researched areas were symptoms, nursing issues, psychosocial issues, cancer services, and experiences of patients, nurses, and caregivers. Although pain and fatigue were studied, many symptoms, such as infection, sleep, wound care, diarrhea, and mouth care, were studied infrequently. Many of the studies reviewed were lacking rigor and had inadequate theoretic explanations. Although the United States contributed the most articles reviewed, Sweden, Finland, and Norway had far more articles when population was factored in. In subjects who had the most common cancers—lung, colorectal, and prostate—a minimal number of studies were found. A review of studies examining the needs of older patients who have cancer when communicating with health care professionals about their treatment found no studies that focused on the needs of older patients, despite the increased incidence of cancer in that population [5].

Failures

Cancer has replaced heart disease as the number 1 killer of Americans under 85 [6]. In 2007, 1,444,920 new cases of cancer were expected to occur in

Americans, and 559,650 are expected to die, more than 1500 people a day [7]. Although great advances have been made in genetics and molecular biology and in cure of cancers, such as some leukemias and lymphomas, a substantial reduction in death rates for most of the common cancers has not occurred [6,8,9]. Health disparities continue to be a major problem within the United States. African Americans are more likely to develop and die from cancer than any other group of people, and death rates from cancer are almost 40% higher for African American men than white men [7]. African Americans have higher mortality rates than whites for all of the major cancer sites (colorectal, lung, breast, and prostate). Minority populations face obstacles in accessing cancer prevention and screening activities and in receiving standard treatment. Poverty, older age, and geographic locale all negatively influence the cancer care a person receives [7].

Many African Americans, the elderly, and those living in medically underserved areas have poor access to quality cancer care [10]. Rural communities often have limited access to quality cancer care. Urban communities, however, where many minorities reside, have shortages of health care professionals. An analysis of physician visits by elderly Medicare beneficiaries found that African Americans were treated by physicians who were less likely to be board certified, and those physicians had difficulties obtaining specialty care for their patients [11].

Because of the endemic nature of hepatitis B infection in Asia, liver cancer is more common there and in recent immigrants. Compared with other Asians, Chinese and Vietnamese women have high incidence and death rates from lung cancer, even with low rates of smoking.

Poverty is a significant negative for people who have cancer and is associated with poorer cancer outcomes regardless of ethnicity [12,13]. People who do not have health insurance and those on Medicaid are more likely to be diagnosed with advanced stages of cancer than their peers who have private health insurance. Five-year survival rates from cancer are 10% lower for those living in poverty [14].

Obesity is a significant risk factor for cancer [15,16]. A significant association exists between body mass index and mortality from most forms of cancer [17]. Those persons who have body mass indices of at least 40 had death rates from all cancers that were 52% higher for men and 62% for women compared with persons of normal weight. Maintaining a healthy body mass index is one of the major lifestyle recommendations shown to reduce cancer risk [18]. Other recommendations include daily physical activity, avoidance of junk food and processed meats, and limiting consumption of red meat and dietary supplements. Obesity rates have increased substantially between 1990 and 2004 [3]. Obesity has adversely affected the incidence of breast cancer, with weight gain and excess adiposity significant risk factors for postmenopausal breast cancer [3]. All of this evidence has stimulated little research activity in prevention of cancer by weight control. There are no randomized clinical trials testing the effect of weight loss on recurrence or survival in obese cancer patients. In a literature search for scientific papers on obesity and cancer over the past 5 years, 2911 articles were found. Of those, 49 were nursing related, published in nursing journals or those having nursing in the title. Six of those 49 were research studies.

Perhaps even more disheartening is the ineffective symptom management and palliative care that many patients who have cancer receive. Studies have shown that pain is inadequately treated in a number of populations, especially minority groups [19,20]. Pain is one of the most common complaints of patients admitted to hospitals, and moderate to severe pain is reported throughout treatment and even after discharge [21]. State policies can promote or interfere in pain management. Some states have intractable pain treatment acts, which are intended to improve pain management by granting physicians immunity from sanctions for prescribing opioids to patients who have such pain problems. Many of these acts, however, imposed more restrictions on opioids prescriptions and do not improve access to pain management care [21]. A study of pharmacies in nonwhite neighborhoods of New York City demonstrated that more than 50% did not have medications stocked to treat severe pain [22]. An examination of state laws and regulations on pain management policies showed several outdated medical concepts and prescribing restrictions and that they did not contain regulations that would make pain management a priority for licensed health care professionals [21].

The American Cancer Society established a goal in 1998 to decrease cancer mortality by 25% by 2015. A midpoint assessment, however, showed the pace of incidence reduction was only half that necessary to achieve the 25% cancer incidence reduction [3]. Cancer incidence rates declined by approximately 0.6% per year between 1992 and 2004. Reduction in cancer incidence was observed in cancers of the prostate, lung in men, colorectum, ovary, oral cavity, stomach, and cervix, and incidence rates have increased for melanoma and cancers of the kidney, liver, thyroid, and esophagus. Little change was seen in incidence of multiple myeloma, non-Hodgkin's lymphoma, leukemia, or cancers of the bladder, brain, or pancreas.

Where to go from here

Although nursing research has addressed some of the concerns and problems afflicting persons who have cancer, it is unclear if any of that research reaches nurses at the bedside. A troubling study on use of evidence in nursing practice states that although nurses often need information for practice, often at least weekly, they are not confident in using databases [23]. The majority of respondents (760 registered nurses) had never sought the help of a hospital librarian or never received instruction in the use of electronic resources. Nurses identified a lack of value for research in practice. Clearly, educators are not reaching students on the importance of research in practice and how to obtain it. With study results such as these, one cannot assume that patients are receiving nursing care that is based on current nursing research. Developing strategies for bringing research to practicing nurses is a priority for the future.

Research is needed in many areas. Lacking in entirety from the nursing literature is any examination of the role of environmental exposures in the development of cancer. These exposures may result in genetic changes and affect patient survival and well-being. Evidence-based cancer prevention strategies must continue to be explored and modifiable risk factors, such as obesity and tobacco cessation, could be major areas of nursing research. Intervention studies that compare factors influencing cancer outcomes, including behavioral and social factors, are needed. Policy is needed to address the major health disparities in cancer care that exist in this country. Transdisciplinary research, which can examine interactions between key variables, such as health literacy and cancer outcomes, also are needed. In summary, the War on Cancer has not been won. Advances have been made, but there is much work to be done.

References

[1] DeVita V. A perspective on the war on cancer. Cancer J 2002;8(5):353–6.

[2] Bach P. Why we'll never cure cancer. Wall Street Journal, October 27, 2007. p. A9. Available at: http://online.wsj.com/article/SB119344360505573496.html. Accessed October 29, 2007.

[3] Sedjo R, Byers T, Barrera E, et al. A midpoint assessment of the American Cancer Society challenge goal to decrease cancer incidence by 25% between 1992 and 2015. CA Cancer J Clin 2007;57(6):326–40.

[4] Molassiotis A, Gibson F, Kelly D, et al. A systematic review of worldwide cancer nursing research: 1994–2003. Cancer Nurs 2006;29(6):431–40.

[5] Jansen J, van Weert J, van Dulmen S, et al. Patient education about treatment in cancer care. Cancer Nurs 2007;30(4):251–9.

[6] Leaf C, Burke D. Why we're losing the war on cancer (and how to win it). Fortune 2004;149: 76–97.

[7] American Cancer Society. Cancer facts and figures 2007. Atlanta (GA): American Cancer Society; 2007.

[8] Bailar J, Gornik H. Cancer undefeated. N Engl J Med 1997;336(22):1569–74.

[9] Sporn M. The War on Cancer: a review. Lancet 1996;347(9012):1377–81.

[10] Underwood S, Powe B, Canales M, et al. Cancer in US ethnic and racial minority populations. Annu Rev Nurs Res 2004;22:217–63.

[11] Bach P, Pham H, Schrag D, et al. Primary care physicians who treat blacks and whites. N Engl J Med 2004;351:575–84.

[12] Muss H. Factors used to select adjuvant therapy of breast cancer in the United States: an overview of age, race and socioeconomic status. J Natl Cancer Inst 2001;30:52–5.

[13] Wrigley H, Roderick P, George S, et al. Inequalities in survival from colorectal cancer: a comparison of the impact of deprivation, treatment and host factors on observed and cause specific survival. J Epidemiol Community Health 2003;57:301–9.

[14] Ward E, Jemal A, Cokkinides V, et al. Cancer disparities by race/ethnicity and socioeconomic status. CA Cancer J Clin 2004;54:78–93.

[15] Hu F, Willett W, Li T, et al. Adiposity as compared with physical activity in predicting mortality among women. N Engl J Med 2004;351:2694–703.

[16] Lippman S, Levin B. Cancer prevention: strong science and real medicine. J Clin Oncol 2005; 23(2):249–53.

[17] Calle E, Rodriguez C, Walker-Thurmond K, et al. Overweight, obesity and mortality from cancer in a prospectively studied cohort of US adults. N Engl J Med 2003;348:1625–38.

[18] World Cancer Research Fund, American Institute for Cancer Research. Food, nutrition, physical activity and the prevention of cancer: a global perspective. Washington, DC: American Institute of Cancer Research; 2007.

[19] Cleeland C, Gonin R, Baez L, et al. Pain and treatment of pain in minority patients with cancer: the Eastern Cooperative Oncology Group minority outpatient pain study. Ann Intern Med 1997;127:813–6.

[20] McDonald D. Gender and ethnic stereotyping and narcotic analgesic administration. Res Nurs Health 1994;17:45–9.

[21] Gilson A, Joranson D, Maurer M. Improving state pain policies: recent progress and continuing opportunities. CA Cancer J Clin 2007;57(6):341–53.

[22] Morrison R, Wallenstein S, Natale D, et al. "We don't carry that"—failure of pharmacies in predominantly nonwhite neighborhoods to stock opioid analgesics. N Engl J Med 2000; 342(14):1023–6.

[23] Pravikoff D, Tanner A, Pierce S. Readiness of US nurses for evidence based practice. Am J Nurs 2005;105(9):40–9.

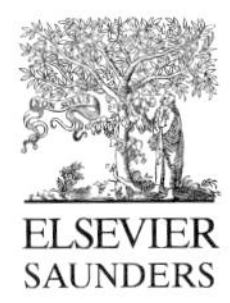
ELSEVIER
SAUNDERS

Nurs Clin N Am 43 (2008) 283–306

NURSING CLINICS OF NORTH AMERICA

Cancer Screening in Men

Thomas J. Gates, MD*, Matthew J. Beelen, MD, Curtis L. Hershey, MD

Department of Family and Community Medicine, Lancaster General Hospital, 555 North Duke Street, Lancaster, PA 17604, USA

Of the 558 million office visits to primary care physicians in 2002, an estimated 23.3%, or 130 million visits, were for preventive care [1]. Although no specific data exist, presumably a high proportion of these visits included at least a discussion of cancer screening and prevention. Thus, cancer screening is one of the most common requests directed to primary care physicians in the office setting. Nevertheless, considerable uncertainty and controversy surround current recommendations for cancer screening [2].

There is good reason to believe that the experience of cancer screening is different for men and women. For at least the past two generations, young women have been socialized to expect Papanicolaou (pap) smears for the detection of cervical cancer as a routine part of their health care, often starting in the teenage years and repeated annually. Most women will know someone who has had an abnormal pap smear requiring follow-up colposcopy, biopsy, and even treatment for a possibly pre-cancerous condition. Furthermore, screening for cervical cancer by pap smears is a prime example of a successful screening program, with mortality rates from cervical cancer declining by at least 60% wherever pap screening has been introduced [3]. Thus, the majority of women come to accept the potential value of cancer screening from a relatively young age. Building on this foundation, mammography screening for breast cancer (although not without controversy) has been an accepted and widely available part of women's health care for at least the past 30 years, often starting by age 40. As with pap smears, many middle aged women will know a friend or relative who has had detection of an early breast cancer, and who will believe that her life has been saved by mammography. In a recent national telephone survey, 99% of

A version of this article was previously published in the March 2006 issue of Primary Care: Clinics in Office Practice.

* Corresponding author.

E-mail address: tjgates@lancastergeneral.org (T.J. Gates).

doi:10.1016/j.cnur.2008.03.004 ***nursing.theclinics.com***

women aged 40 and older reported ever having had a pap test, and 89% have had mammography [4].

By contrast, men may have less reason to feel positively about cancer screening. The most important cause of cancer mortality in men (as for women) is lung cancer, but early efforts to screen for this condition with annual chest x-rays and sputum cytology were disappointing, and are no longer recommended [5]. Prostate cancer is the second most common cause of cancer mortality in men, but PSA screening remains mired in controversy more than 10 years after it was first recommended as a screening test. Screening for colon cancer (the third most common cause of cancer mortality in men), although promising, is a relatively new recommendation.

In this article, we look at current recommendations, evidence for, and controversy surrounding screening for cancers of the lung, colon, and prostate, which together account for 51% of cancer deaths in men (Table 1). We also look at screening for testicular cancer, which, although a relatively minor contributor to cancer mortality, is a prototypically male cancer with a proposed screening test. Other causes of cancer mortality in men are important (Table 1), but with no generally accepted screening tests available, are outside the scope of this article.

Screening, because it involves asymptomatic patients, occupies a unique place in the practice of medicine. To better understand specific recommendations and current controversies, we turn first to a consideration of the "basic science" of screening.

General considerations in screening

Screening can be defined as the application of diagnostic tests or procedures to asymptomatic people for the purpose of dividing them into two

Table 1
Estimated incidence and mortality of selected cancers in US males, 2005

Estimated new cases of cancer	Total 710,040	Estimated cancer deaths	Total 295,280
Prostate	33%	Lung	31%
Lung	13%	Prostate	10%
Colorectal	10%	Colorectal	10%
Bladder	7%	Pancreas	5%
Melanoma	5%	Leukemia	4%
Lymphoma	4%	Esophagus	4%
Kidney	3%	Liver	3%
Leukemia	3%	Lymphoma	3%
Oral cavity	3%	Bladder	3%
Pancreas	2%	Kidney	3%
All other sites	17%	All other sites	24%

Data from Jemal A, Murray T, Ward E, et al. Cancer statistics, 2005. CA Cancer J Clin 2005;55:10–30.

groups: those who have a condition that would benefit from early intervention, and those who do not [6]. For both patients and clinicians, the value of screening is often taken as self-evident: it is good to detect disease earlier rather than later, when it is potentially more amenable to treatment and potential cure. However, it is important to recognize that the ultimate purpose of screening is to reduce morbidity and mortality. Early detection by itself does not justify screening, but only early detection that in turn leads to a measurable improvement in outcomes [2].

The seemingly self-evident value of screening is reflected in a nearly insatiable enthusiasm for cancer screening on the part of the public. In a national telephone survey, 87% of US adults believe that routine cancer screening is "almost always a good idea," and 74% believe that finding cancer early saves lives "most" or "all of the time." A substantial majority of respondents felt it would be "irresponsible" for a 55-year-old in average health to forego available screening (from 54% to 79%, depending on the test); 86% of respondents said that they would want a total-body computed tomography (CT) scan, and 85% of those said they would choose such a scan rather than receiving $1000 in cash [4].

Faced with this public enthusiasm for screening, it is sometimes difficult for clinicians to look objectively at the evidence for cancer screening, which in general shows a mortality benefit much more modest than the public perception [7]. Primary care practitioners, like the public, certainly place high value on the early detection and treatment of cancer, but this needs to be balanced by other values, such as avoiding ineffective interventions, the duty not to harm patients, and the efficient use of scarce societal resources.

By definition, screening tests are applied to asymptomatic patients, and hidden within this medical encounter with an asymptomatic patient is a subtle but important shift in the doctor–patient relationship. In ordinary clinical practice, the patient initiates the encounter because of a troubling symptom: the patient is asking for help in understanding and treating the symptom or disease in question. The physician pledges to help, but can make no guarantee, because the troubling symptom may point to a condition beyond the ability of current medical practice to cure.

By contrast, the screening encounter is usually initiated by the physician (or indirectly, by professional or advocacy groups that have convinced the patient to seek screening). In this situation, a proposal to screen a healthy asymptomatic person involves an "implied promise": not just that the screening test seems like a good idea, but that it is in fact beneficial, that it will do more good than harm [8,9]. This introduces an often-neglected ethical dimension to screening [8,10,11]. Because any proposed screening procedure involves potential harm to an asymptomatic patient (as opposed to a patient seeking relief from symptoms), principles of patient autonomy and informed consent would seem to be especially compelling. The first principle of screening is that whereas it is by definition impossible to make an asymptomatic patient feel better, it is quite possible to make the patient feel worse.

Benefits and harms of screening

As in all of medicine, the decision to screen rests on the balance of benefits and harms. The benefits of screening would seem to be self-evident: early detection, with improved outcomes, and higher cure rates. However, the benefit of screening is entirely dependent on one key assumption: that treatment initiated during an early asymptomatic period of the disease will yield better outcomes than treatment which is initiated at a later period, when the disease has become symptomatic. Clearly, this assumption is not always true.

To illustrate this point, Figure 1 shows the schematic natural history of a hypothetical disease. The "critical point" is that point in the natural history before which therapy is relatively effective, and after which it is relatively ineffective [9]. In the case of cancer, the critical point can be thought of as the time at which regional or distant metastasis occurs. Whether a specific cancer is amenable to screening depends largely on when in the natural history the critical point occurs. If the critical point is early, as with lung cancer, screening will be ineffective; if it is late, as with uterine cancer, screening will be unnecessary. In reality, the situation is even more complicated, because any given type of cancer can have a spectrum of presentations, from aggressive and already metastasized when detected by screening, to indolent and still curable even when clinically advanced [2,7].

Even if a screening test has proven benefits, those benefits accrue only to a few individuals. By contrast, all individuals participating in a screening program are at risk for adverse consequence [8]. Over and above the cost and discomfort of the test, the most common adverse consequence is a false-positive result. Because the diseases being screened for have a low prevalence, then by Baye's theorem any positive result on a screening test will have a low positive predictive value (often approximately 10% to 20%).

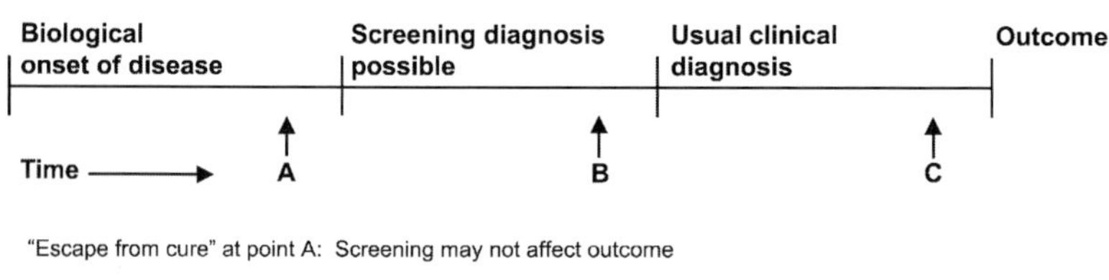

"Escape from cure" at point A: Screening may not affect outcome

"Escape from cure" at point B: High priority for screening

"Escape from cure" at point C: Education and improved access to care may be more efficient than screening tests

Fig. 1. Relationship of natural history of disease, critical point, and screening, (*From* Goroll AH, May LA, Mulley AG Jr, editors. Primary Care Medicine: office evaluation and management of the adult patient. 4th edition. Philadelphia: Lippincott Williams & Wilkins; 2000. p. 15; with permission.)

As a consequence, most positive results will be false-positives, leading to further work-up, added costs, and patient anxiety (e.g., a negative prostate biopsy result after an elevated screening PSA test). Related to a false-positive test is the harm of overdiagnosis: the detection by screening of "pseudodisease," or disease that is present on biopsy but that is not destined to produce significant clinical disease during the lifetime of the patient [12], either because it is very indolent or because competing causes of mortality limit life expectancy. Overdiagnosis can lead to unnecessary treatment and resulting morbidity and mortality (e.g., incontinence and impotence after a radical prostatectomy for an asymptomatic low-grade prostate cancer detected on PSA screening).

False-negative results can also be harmful, by providing false reassurance and thereby encouraging patients to neglect important symptoms or risky behavior (e.g., a negative chest x-ray in a smoker, who then decides to continue to smoke). Finally, a screening test may be completely accurate in diagnosing a disease, but if the subsequent therapy is either ineffective or toxic, then the patient has been harmed rather than helped [9] (e.g., a post-operative death after radical prostatectomy done for asymptomatic prostate cancer detected by screening).

In light of these potential harms to healthy patients, justification for a screening test requires a more rigorous standard of effectiveness than is usual in ordinary clinical practice. In fact, one of the important historical roots of evidence-based medicine was in the evaluation of screening tests, as pioneered by Frame and Carlson [13], and subsequently developed by the Canadian Task Force on the Periodic Health Exam [14] and the US Preventive Services Task Force [15]. Based on their work, and recalling that early detection by itself does not justify screening, Box 1 describes the necessary characteristics of a successful screening program.

Bias in the evaluation of screening tests

Evaluation of screening tests is complicated by certain biases, which occur because screening tests alter the natural history of the disease in question. All forms of bias tend to make screening initially appear more effective than it really is, so failure to account for them may cause both patients and physicians to overestimate the benefit of screening.

Figure 2 illustrates the important concept of lead-time bias, which occurs when we neglect to account for the asymptomatic period in the natural history. Patients with cancer diagnosed by screening always have a longer survival after diagnosis, but this may not be because they are actually living longer, but because they found out about their diagnosis at an earlier point in the natural history [9]. Surrogate measures like median survival or 5-year survival depend on the elapsed time from diagnosis to death and are therefore subject to lead-time bias. Consequently, the only way to avoid lead-time bias is to compare actual mortality rates in a screened and unscreened population.

Box 1. Criteria for screening

Characteristics of the disease:

- Significant impact on the quality or length of life
- Acceptable treatment(s) available
- Asymptomatic period during which detection and treatment is feasible
- Treatment initiated during asymptomatic period results in better outcomes than treatment initiated after symptoms appear.

Characteristics of the screening test:

- Sufficiently sensitive to detect asymptomatic disease
- Sufficiently specific to minimize false-positive results
- Acceptable to patients

Characteristics of the screened population:

- Sufficiently high disease prevalence to justify the cost of screening
- Access to relevant medical care
- Willingness to comply with subsequent diagnostic tests and necessary therapy.

Adapted from Mulley AG. Health maintenance and the role of screening. In: Goroll AH, Mulley AG, editors. Primary Care Medicine. 4th edition. Philadelphia: Lipincott Williams & Wilkins; 2000. p. 14.

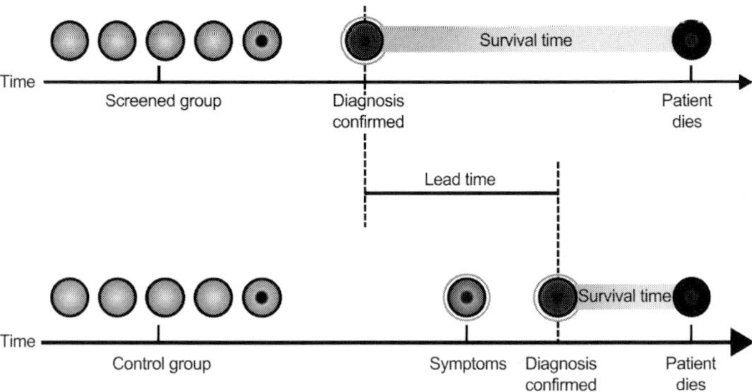

Fig. 2. Lead-time bias. In the example shown, the diagnosis of disease is made earlier in the screened group, resulting in an apparent increase in survival time (lead-time bias), although in reality the time of death is the same in both groups. (*From* Patz EF Jr, Goodman PC, Bepler G. Screening for lung cancer. N Eng J Med 2000;343:1628–9; with permission.)

Length (or length-time) bias, illustrated in Figure 3, occurs because of the heterogeneity of disease, which presents across a broad spectrum of biologic activity. A screening program may appear to improve survival when in fact it has only preferentially selected out the subgroup with the best prognosis [9]. Because of length-time bias, it is important that screening tests be evaluated by population-based randomized controlled trials, rather than a simple comparison of tumors detected by screening versus those presenting clinically.

Figure 4 illustrates overdiagnosis bias, which occurs when a sensitive screening test is able to diagnose pathology that is real but clinically insignificant. When overdiagnosis occurs, the screened group will have a much lower case fatality rate, even in the absence of any therapy, because the clinically insignificant cases artificially increase the denominator in the screened group. Overdiagnosis is likely to be a factor in both PSA screening and CT screening for lung cancer.

Selection (or screening) bias occurs because people who volunteer for screening tend to be healthier than those who do not volunteer, with lower mortality not just from the disease in question but also from all causes of mortality. Therefore, people who volunteer for screening should not be compared with a non-volunteer control group, but instead populations should be randomized to screening or control arms. Even in randomized trials, those who comply with screening are healthier and have lower all-cause mortality than those who do not comply, so bias can be avoided only when data is subject to "intention-to-treat" analysis. Without the safeguards of randomization and intention-to-treat analysis, any observed benefit may

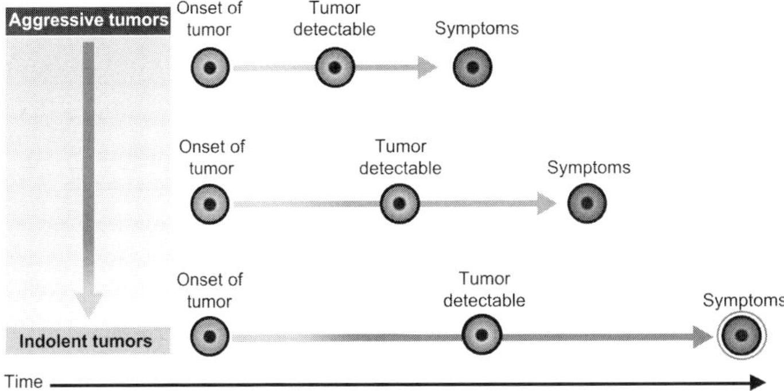

Fig. 3. Length-time bias. The probability of detecting disease is related to the growth rate of the tumor. Aggressive, rapidly growing tumors have a short potential screening period (the interval between possible detection and the occurrence of symptoms). Thus, unless the screening test is repeated frequently, patients with aggressive tumors are less likely to be detected when they are asymptomatic. As a result, a higher proportion of indolent tumors is found in the screened group, causing an apparent improvement in survival. (*From* Patz EF Jr, Goodman PC, Bepler G. Screening for lung cancer. N Eng J Med 2000;343:1628–9; with permission.)

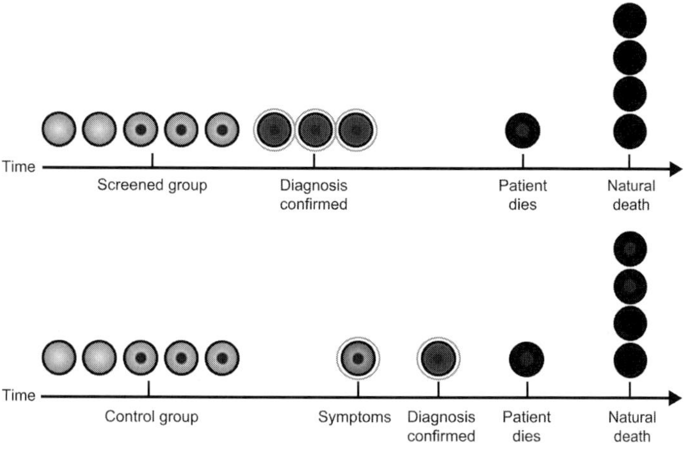

Fig. 4. Overdiagnosis bias. Overdiagnosis bias is an extreme form of length-time bias. The detection of very indolent tumors in the screened group produces apparent increases in the number of cases of cancer (three in the screened group and one in the control group) and in survival (two of three patients in the screened group were treated and died of other causes, without evidence of cancer [66 percent survival]), and the one patient in the control group did not survive [0 percent survival]), with no effect on mortality (one death from cancer in each group). Two patients in the control group died with undiagnosed cancer that did not affect their natural life span. (*From* Patz EF Jr, Goodman PC, Bepler G. Screening for lung cancer. N Eng J Med 2000;343:1628–9; with permission.)

be due not to the screening intervention, but only to the self-selection of a cohort of healthy volunteers [9].

Recently, two new types of bias have been described in relation to the controversy over the proper end-point of a screening trial: disease-specific mortality (which is easier to demonstrate) or all-cause mortality (which is more difficult to demonstrate but less subject to bias) [16]. Assigning a specific cause of death can be subject to bias. For example, a patient with localized lung cancer diagnosed on a screening chest x-ray dies of sudden cardiac death some weeks later. Even though the cause of death was not lung cancer, that diagnosis will often "stick" (so-called sticky-diagnosis bias), thus artificially increasing the disease-specific mortality in the screening group. By contrast, failure to account for adverse effects of screening can bias disease-specific mortality in favor of screening (so-called slippery-linkage bias). For example, a man with an elevated PSA undergoes a biopsy, has localized prostate cancer diagnosed, has a radical prostatectomy, and then 3 weeks later dies of a pulmonary embolus. He did not die of prostate cancer, and yet he may well have died of *screening* for prostate cancer.

All-cause mortality is not affected by either sticky-diagnosis bias or slippery-linkage bias, and thus theoretically provides a less biased measure of the true effects of screening on mortality. In practice, however, a decrease in all-cause mortality may be an impossibly high standard by which to judge screening interventions (especially for low-prevalence diseases), and would require a sample size at least an order of magnitude greater than previous screening trials [17,18]. In the absence of trials large enough to detect a decrease in all-cause mortality, the best we can do may be to design trials that minimize any bias in assignment of the cause of death.

Evaluation of screening tests

Because of the complex and unpredictable effect of these various types of bias, the only reliable way to prove the effectiveness of a screening program is to demonstrate lower mortality (all-cause or, more commonly, disease-specific) in a randomly assigned screened population, compared with unscreened controls, using intention-to-treat analysis, a so-called randomized controlled trial (RCT) [9]. Screening interventions that have not fulfilled this high standard of evidence should be considered experimental, with unproven benefits, and patients should give informed consent before participating [8,10].

Even when screening tests have fulfilled this high standard of evidence, the manner in which results are reported can influence our perception of the magnitude of the benefit [19]. In general, describing a screening test in terms of the relative risk reduction is subjectively heard by most people as the most favorable interpretation of the same data. For example, "mammography reduces breast cancer mortality by 25%" sounds more effective than "one breast cancer death is prevented for every thousand women screened." There is an increasing tendency in the literature to evaluate screening tests in terms of the number needed to screen (NNS), which is calculated simply as the reciprocal of the absolute risk reduction (ARR) (NNS = 1/ARR) [20,21]. The NNS represents the number of *patients* who would need to be screened over a given time period (usually 5 or 10 years) to prevent one death from the disease in question. (The number of screening *tests* that would be required to prevent that one death would be up to 10-times higher, depending on the frequency of screening.) The NNS reflects both the prevalence of the disease and the effectiveness of therapy, and has the advantage of being easy to calculate and intuitively useful to both clinicians and patients. It does not, however, specifically account for either the risks or costs of screening.

Ideally, all screening tests would have an agreed on NNS. However, to calculate a NNS, the absolute risk reduction (derived from a properly conducted RCT) must be known. In reality, of the specific cancer screening tests to which we now turn, such trials have been conducted only for fecal occult blood testing to screen for colon cancer. This unfortunate deficit in our understanding results in significant uncertainty surrounding most screening tests for cancer.

Epidemiology of cancer in men

Cancer is the second leading cause of mortality among US men, accounting for 24.1% of all male deaths in 2002, compared with 28.4% of deaths from heart disease. However, in those younger than age 80 (98% of the population), cancer has now surpassed heart disease as the leading cause of mortality. Of almost 800,000 total deaths in men younger than age 80 in 2002, 26.9% (214,929 deaths) were caused by cancer, and 25.5% (203,992) were caused by heart disease. Age adjusted cancer death rates have declined by 1.5% per year from 1993 to 2001, but the death rate from heart disease has declined much more drastically (nearly 50% in the past 30 years) [22].

In men, cancers of the lung, prostate, and colon together account for 51% of all cancer deaths (Table 1). We turn now to consideration of screening for these specific cancers, plus the unique issue of screening for testicular cancer.

Testicular cancer

Because cancer of the testicle affects primarily young men, it can be seen as analogous to cancer of the cervix in women. However, screening for testicular cancer has not gained widespread attention or acceptance, for two key reasons. First, testicular cancer has a relatively low incidence. With an estimated 8010 new cases diagnosed in 2005, testicular cancer only accounts for 1.1% of cancers in men [22]. Second, testicular cancer is highly treatable even after symptoms develop. An estimated 390 men will die of this disease in the US in 2005 [22]. Five-year survival is well over 90% with current treatment regimens [23].

Based on these favorable aspects of testicular cancer and the paucity of data to support generalized screening in asymptomatic men, the USPSTF recommends against routine screening (D recommendation). There is no evidence that either clinical examination or testicular self-examination reduces mortality from testicular cancer. Furthermore, because of its low incidence and favorable outcome, no such evidence is likely to be forthcoming. The USPSTF therefore concluded that the harms of generalized screening outweigh the benefits [23].

However, some have recommended screening in certain high-risk populations, including men with cryptorchidism, testicular atrophy, or ambiguous genitalia. The Canadian Task Force on Preventive Health Care (CTFPHC) contends that although there is insufficient evidence to make a formal recommendation, individuals with these risk factors should undergo regular physician examinations [24]. The American Cancer Society is more specific, stating that high-risk patients should have monthly examinations [25]. The USPSTF does not make a recommendation regarding screening in higher risk patients.

In the absence of recommendations to screen low-risk men for testicular cancer, it seems prudent for physicians to encourage "testicular awareness." For example, during the inguinal examination as part of a pre-participation or driver's physical, the physician can simply state that although testicular cancer is not common, it is an important cause of cancer in young men, and that should he ever notice an unusual or painless lump in or near his testicle, he should have it promptly checked by a physician.

Colorectal cancer

Screening for colorectal cancer is of interest to us from two perspectives. First, it is the only major cancer occurring in both men and women that has an accepted screening strategy, thereby allowing for direct comparison of compliance between the sexes (although in fact data are hard to come by). Second, because of very favorable biological characteristics (a known precancerous lesion with a long asymptomatic period, and dramatically improved outcomes when detected and treated early), colorectal cancer should in theory be very amenable to successful screening. A number of different options for screening have been proposed, but at this point the only strategy shown to lower colorectal cancer mortality in prospective RCTs is screening with fecal occult blood testing (FOBT).

A recent Cochrane Review summarized the use FOBT in the prevention of colorectal cancer mortality. Six trials involving 442,000 patients were included, and showed a combined relative risk of colorectal cancer mortality of 0.84 (95% CI: 0.77–0.92) in the screened group [26], and a NNS of 1237 patients (CI, 782–2961) to prevent one colon cancer death over 8 to 13 years [27].

Other screening strategies have also been advocated, most prominently flexible sigmoidoscopy (either alone or in combination with FOBT) and colonoscopy. To date, there have been no prospective RCTs evaluating the effect of either of these modalities on colorectal cancer mortality, nor have there been any direct comparisons between different screening strategies. In the absence of direct data, two cost-effectiveness studies based on economic models have suggested that colonoscopy is a reasonable screening procedure, with the marginal cost per year of life saved comparable to other accepted screening procedures [28,29].

The argument in favor of colonoscopy as a primary screening modality is its presumed high sensitivity for significant lesions throughout the entire colon. A Veterans Administration study demonstrated that in asymptomatic patients undergoing colonoscopy, the sensitivity of the 60-cm sigmoidoscope for advanced colonic neoplasia would have been only 70.3%, increasing to 75.8% with the addition of FOBT, compared with colonoscopy [30]. In this population, with a 10.6% prevalence of advanced colonic neoplasia, the negative predictive value of a normal sigmoidoscopy combined with a negative FOBT was 97%.

In 2002, the USPSTF issued revised recommendations on screening for colorectal cancer, accompanied by a thorough review of the relevant literature. They found good evidence that screening for colorectal cancer reduces disease-specific mortality, and endorsed screening for patients 50 years and older (A level recommendation). They found insufficient data to determine which screening strategy is most effective. Specifically, they concluded that "it is unclear whether the increased accuracy of colonoscopy compared with alternative screening methods offsets the procedure's additional complications, inconvenience, and costs" [31]. Thus, the Task Force strongly endorses colorectal cancer screening but does not endorse a specific or single strategy. According to both the USPSTF and the American Cancer Society, acceptable strategies, depending on patient preference and local resources, would include: annual FOBT; sigmoidoscopy every 5 years; annual FOBT plus sigmoidoscopy every 5 years; double contrast barium enema every 5 years; and colonoscopy every 10 years [31,32].

Although colonoscopy clearly has the highest sensitivity of any of the screening strategies, widespread implementation of screening colonoscopy faces three unresolved issues: the systems issue of whether there are a sufficient number of trained endoscopists to perform the required colonoscopies; the economic issue of the high total cost (especially with studies so far unable to demonstrate a decline in all-cause mortality with screening); and the ethical issue of possible harm, particularly the small but real possibility of colonic perforation. Because of these potential problems, there is ongoing interest in new technologies for colorectal cancer screening. Of these, noninvasive CT colonography (so-called virtual colonoscopy) shows the most promise.

CT colonography technology is rapidly evolving, and two recent reports give somewhat contradictory assessments of its suitability as a screening strategy. In the first and more favorable report, 1233 asymptomatic adults underwent same-day CT colonography followed by conventional colonoscopy (initially blinded to the results of the CT colonoscopy, but then segmentally unblinded and compared with the CT colonography; the unblinded colonoscopy was considered the "gold standard"). Surprisingly, they found that CT colonography was actually more sensitive than conventional colonoscopy (93.9% versus 91.5% for the presence of polyps at least 8 mm in diameter). Using a strategy of screening CT colonography for everyone and referral of only those patients with apparent polyps 8 mm or larger for same-day colonoscopy, only 13.5% of patients would have required conventional colonoscopy, and the negative predictive value of a normal CT study exceeded 99% [33].

A second study gave much less promising results. Using a similar methodology, 615 patients referred for clinically indicated colonoscopy underwent CT colonography followed by blinded and then segmentally unblinded colonoscopy. The sensitivity for detection of polyps at least 10 mm in diameter was a disappointing 55% (compared with 99% for colonoscopy) [34]. The difference in the two studies can be attributed partly to a difference in the technology used and possibly a difference in the experience of the radiologists, but partly remains unexplained. It seems reasonable to conclude that screening with CT colonography is not yet ready for wide application, but that as the technology improves and experience increases, it may at some point in the future provide a reasonable alternative to conventional colonoscopy.

Despite evidence indicating that screening for colorectal cancer saves lives, there is ample indication that compliance with recommendations for colorectal cancer screening is lower than for other cancers. In a comprehensive review of barriers to colorectal cancer screening, Wender states that fewer than 40% of adults older than age 50 have ever been screened, and less than 30% are up to date with colon cancer screening [35]. In the CDC's comprehensive Behavioral Risk Factor Surveillance Survey (2002), the prevalence of recent cancer screening (as defined by accepted guidelines for each cancer) was 41% for endoscopy for colon cancer, compared with 55% for PSA screening for prostate cancer, 61% for mammography for breast cancer, and 88% for pap tests for cervical cancer [32].

Data on the comparative compliance of men versus women are somewhat contradictory. In a telephone survey of a representative sample, 60% of women versus 50% of men 50 and older had received endoscopic screening for colorectal cancer, but this difference did not quite achieve statistical significance.(Steven Woloshin, M.D., personal communication, December 14, 2004). In the one trial of FOBT that reported compliance in men versus women, women had higher compliance rates in all age cohorts younger than age 65, but after 65 men and women had identical compliance [36]. A French trial showed consistently higher compliance with FOBT among women compared with men, through five rounds of screening [37]. A large retrospective chart audit showed that in patients 50 and older, a slightly higher proportion of women than men had received FOBT within the past year (28% versus 26%), but more men than women had received flexible sigmoidoscopy within the previous 5 years (22% versus 17%) [38]. Similarly, the Massachusetts Behavioral Risk Factor Surveillance System documented that women were more likely to have had FOBT alone (27% versus 17%), but men were more likely to have had flexible sigmoidoscopy (75% versus 63%) [39]. By contrast, in actual clinical practice, women may underestimate their risk for colorectal cancer, and some have suggested that clinicians may fail to offer screening (especially sigmoidoscopy) to women at the same rate as men [35,40].

Perhaps more important than differences in compliance between men and women is the overall poor compliance with colorectal cancer screening recommendations in all demographic categories. In Wender's detailed description of the many barriers to colorectal cancer screening, he draws attention to one factor related to gender roles and advocacy: "Breast cancer is a women's issue. Prostate cancer is a men's issue. Until recently, colon cancer was no one's issue. This lack of ownership limits patient demand and advocacy" [35].

Lung cancer

After years of relative quiet, screening for lung cancer is once again becoming a topic of contentious debate within the screening community, as some believe that new technology has finally made screening feasible. The debate is important, because lung cancer is by far the most common cause of cancer mortality in the US, accounting for 31% of all cancer deaths in men. In 2005, lung cancer will cause an estimated 90,490 deaths in US males, more than three times the number of deaths from either prostate or colon cancer [22].

Proposals to screen for lung cancer using either chest radiography or sputum cytology date back to the 1950s, with several early reports indicating such screening led to a shift to earlier stage disease and improved 5-year survival rates [5]. These favorable results led the American Cancer Society to advocate annual screening chest radiographs for smokers. Subsequently, several large RCTs (summarized in a recent Cochrane Review of seven studies with 245,000 subjects) showed that there was no decrease in lung cancer mortality in intensively screened subjects, compared with less intensively screened controls [41,42]. In retrospect, the favorable early results probably were caused by length-time and lead-time bias. Lung cancer would seem to represent the prototype of a disease where the critical point of regional and distant metastasis occurs very early in the natural history of the disease, so that no screening modality is likely to be effective [2]. The American Cancer Society withdrew its recommendation for screening chest x-rays in 1980, and since then no authoritative organization has recommended screening for lung cancer by chest x-ray or sputum cytology.

Over the past few years, remarkable advances in the technology of low-dose computerized tomography (LDCT) have begun to erode the prevailing pessimism concerning screening for lung cancer. Early reports of promising results came from Japan, but in the US enthusiasm for CT screening dates to the initial publication of results from the Early Lung Cancer Action Project (ELCAP) in 1999. A cohort of 1000 volunteers at risk for lung cancer underwent both chest x-ray and LDCT. 27 lung cancers were detected, of which 26 were resectable and 23 (85%) were stage I. Compared with chest x-ray, LDCT detected three times as many non-calcified nodules, four times as many lung cancers, and six times as many stage I (potentially curable) cancers [43]. However, there was no control group that did not receive LDCT, so no conclusions about mortality can be drawn from this study.

A similar cohort study from the Mayo Clinic demonstrates some of the potential problems with LDCT screening. Of the 1520 subjects who underwent three annual LDCT screening examinations, fully 69% had findings of one or more uncalcified nodules, therefore requiring further testing (the comparable yield in the ELCAP cohort was 23%). Ultimately, only 1.3% of these nodules proved to be malignant, for a false-positive rate approaching 99%. Ultimately, LDCT led to a diagnosis of lung cancer in 2.4% of the cohort, comparable to the ELCAP study; 60% of the non-small cell cancers detected were stage IA [44]. In their discussion, the authors expressed concern about the possibility of overdiagnosis, the high rate of false-positives, financial and emotional costs, potential harm from surgery for benign nodules, and the difficulty of gaining truly informed consent from study subjects.

Based on these and other studies, it now seems incontestable that LDCT scanning can diagnose asymptomatic lung cancer in greater numbers and at an earlier stage than would otherwise be possible. There is preliminary data that the case fatality rate of lung cancer diagnosed by LDCT is as low as 4% [45], compared with 90% in clinically diagnosed lung cancer [46]. However, without mortality data from a RCT, such results could still represent some "combination of selection, length, overdiagnosis, and lead-time biases" [44]. At present, at least three such RCTs have been funded and are enrolling patients, but results are at least a decade away [46]. In the meantime, advocates of CT screening have begun to argue that it is impractical and perhaps unethical to wait for the results of these RCTs, given the favorable preliminary data and the huge public health impact of lung cancer [47,48].

Because of the absence of data demonstrating mortality benefit and the potential harm caused by screening, the USPSTF in its updated 2004 recommendation concluded that there is insufficient evidence to recommend for or against screening for lung cancer (I recommendation). They cited fair evidence that LDCT, and even chest radiography and sputum cytology can detect cancers at an earlier stage, but poor evidence of any mortality benefit. Furthermore, the USPSTF could not determine the balance between the benefit of early detection and the potential for significant harm from diagnostic testing [49].

The American College of Chest Physicians (ACCP) made similar but slightly more specific recommendations in 2003. They recommended against use of chest radiography or sputum cytology in screening asymptomatic individuals (D recommendation). The ACCP also currently recommends against use of either single or serial LDCTs for screening asymptomatic patients, but does recommend informing high-risk patients so that they might consider enrollment in on-going clinical trials [50]. Likewise, the Society of Thoracic Radiology does not advocate screening for lung cancer with CT, except in the setting of controlled clinical trials [51].

Amidst the ongoing debate about the value of screening for early detection of lung cancer, it is important that we not forget that lung cancer, more than any other major cancer, is largely preventable. It is estimated that as many as 87% of lung cancers are attributable to cigarette smoking [46], and the twentieth century epidemic of lung cancer has paralleled the smoking habits of the US population, with a 20-fold increase in mortality rates from lung cancer in US men beginning in approximately 1930 and peaking in approximately 1990, followed by a modest 1.9% per year decline in mortality rates beginning in 1991 [22], reflecting a decline in the percentage of men who smoke [46]. Ultimately, smoking prevention and cessation programs may have a larger impact on lung cancer mortality than any screening program.

Prostate cancer

In many ways, prostate cancer in men parallels breast cancer in women. Both cancers occur largely or exclusively in one sex, and both are the second leading cause of cancer mortality in their respective sexes (behind lung cancer). Breast cancer accounts for approximately 40,000 female deaths per year, and before a recent decline in mortality rates, prostate cancer likewise accounted for about 40,000 deaths per year (now approximately 30,000) [22]. First breast cancer and later prostate cancer have been the target of large public education campaigns (including US Postal Service stamps to raise money for research), and both have had their celebrity advocates. Finally, both prostate cancer and breast cancer are increasing in incidence but decreasing in mortality.

Since the introduction of the prostate-specific antigen (PSA) assay in 1986, the male public has shown an increasing interest in and acceptance of PSA screening, to the point that one could now argue that it has become the standard of care in the United States. A CDC survey in 2002 estimated that 55% of men older than age 50, and 62% of men 65 and older, have had PSA screening within the past year (comparable to mammography rates in women) [32]. In the face of this increasing acceptance of screening, it is important to realize that to date, no RCT has provided evidence that screening for prostate cancer decreases disease-specific mortality. Given these two facts (the lack of evidence for a mortality benefit and the acceptance of PSA screening as the *de facto* standard of care), it is hardly surprising that PSA screening continues to be a subject of controversy and confusion [52,53]. In an attempt to make sense of the current situation, we review important recent epidemiologic trends in prostate cancer, characteristics of the PSA test, current evidence regarding screening, information about strategies that might increase the accuracy of screening, and current recommendations by authorities regarding screening. However, it is important to acknowledge from the beginning that given the uncertain state of our current knowledge, the decision of whether to screen for prostate cancer must ultimately depend on the individual judgment of the physician and patient.

Prostate cancer is the second most common cause of cancer death in men, with 30,000 deaths per year in the United States. However, it is often said that many more men die *with* than *from* prostate cancer. The lifetime risk of developing the disease is approximately 16%, whereas the risk of dying from prostate cancer is 3% [54]. Furthermore, studies suggest that the incidence of histological cancer may be much higher than the incidence of clinical disease, with up to 70% of men age 65 to 80 showing pathological evidence of prostate cancer at autopsy [55]. The gap between the histological and clinical incidence of prostate cancer, as well as the gap between the clinical incidence and mortality rate, both suggest that any screening test which diagnoses asymptomatic prostate cancer may well lead to overdiagnosis, i.e., the diagnosis of disease that is of no clinical significance during the patient's lifetime.

The introduction of PSA testing in 1986 appears to have altered the epidemiology of prostate cancer. Over the first 6 years of the PSA era (1987–1992), the apparent incidence (i.e., the number of cases diagnosed) of prostate cancer nearly doubled, followed by a steep decline from 1992 to 1996. Because PSA screening can detect prostate cancer up to 12 years before it would be clinically diagnosed (lead time) [55], its introduction initially identified a large cohort of men who would have otherwise had the disease diagnosed over the next decade or more, thereby artificially inflating the incidence for the first several years of its availability. Once this cohort was identified by screening, the incidence of prostate cancer fell back toward what it had been before PSA availability. However, since 1997 the incidence has again been increasing, presumably because PSA is sensitive enough to identify a much higher proportion of clinically silent disease than was previously possible. The current incidence of 168 per 100,000 men is well under the peak incidence of 1992, but also well above the incidence of the pre-PSA era [54]. These recent large fluctuations in the incidence of prostate cancer can thus be understood as a predictable consequence of the introduction of a sensitive screening test, rather than to any underlying change in the "real" incidence of the disease.

It is more difficult to dismiss the recent changes in prostate cancer mortality (i.e., the number of men dying from the disease). The age-adjusted mortality rate for prostate cancer has decreased at least 20% since its peak in 1991 [54] and is now falling by 4% per year [22]. For theoretical reasons having to do with the long natural history of the disease, some have argued that the decline in mortality came too soon after the introduction of PSA testing to be attributed entirely to screening [56]. However, improvements in the treatment of advanced prostate cancer are unlikely by themselves to fully account for the fall in mortality. Most of the fall in mortality can be attributed to the well-documented shift toward earlier and more localized disease, with fewer men presenting with distant disease [57]. This stage-shift would seem to argue in favor of screening as the major factor that has led to decreasing mortality.

Despite the suggestive epidemiologic evidence, a mortality benefit from PSA screening has yet to be demonstrated in a RCT. A screening trial from Quebec did suggest a mortality benefit, but it has been criticized for issues of bias and various methodological problems [56]. Likewise, cohort studies in Austria and British Columbia suggest a mortality benefit for screening but results are inconsistent and do not convincingly link screening with decreased mortality [54,56]. Other studies have shown that changes in mortality rates in several countries do not correspond to intensity of screening [57].

Two studies currently in progress should give definitive answers to the mortality question. The Prostate, Lung, Colorectal, and Ovary Trial

(PLCO) in the United States and the European Randomized Study of Screening for Prostate Cancer (ERSPC) in Europe were both designed to find a disease-specific mortality benefit from PSA screening [56]. They will also look at cost-effectiveness and quality-of-life measures. Results are expected by 2008, and will hopefully be able to better guide public policy regarding prostate cancer screening.

Part of the difficulty in evaluating screening for prostate cancer comes from the characteristics of the screening tests themselves. Traditionally, screening was performed by digital rectal examination, but by itself this can miss up to 40% of cancers [58]. The superior sensitivity of PSA screening would seem to be an obvious benefit for detecting early stage prostate cancer. However, the true sensitivity of PSA is difficult to determine, primarily because it would require performing biopsies (the gold standard) on all study subjects, even those with "negative" PSA levels [59]. The sensitivity of PSA will also increase if the threshold for an abnormal level is lowered, but at the cost of increasing false positive results. The most common cutoff used is 4 ng/mL, but it is now clear that many cancers occur in men with PSA levels less than this. In the ERSPC, more than one-third of the cancers were diagnosed in men with PSA levels less than 4 ng/mL [60]. Another recent study, reporting on the results of biopsy samples on a cohort of men who had PSA levels less than 4 ng/mL for 7 years in a row, found that 15% of these men had evidence of prostate cancer on biopsy. For the subgroup whose PSA was between 3.1 and 4.0 ng/mL, the incidence of cancer on biopsy was 26.9% [61]. Thus, it is clear that the conventional cutoff of 4.0 ng/mL misses many cancers, including some that appear to be clinically aggressive.

The specificity of PSA testing is also unknown, but has been estimated to be approximately 60% to 70% [55], meaning that up to 40% of men who do not have prostate cancer will have elevated PSA levels. In addition to prostate cancer, benign prostatic hypertrophy, prostatitis, recent ejaculation, and minor trauma can all elevate PSA levels [59]. The high percentage of false-positives leads to extra cost, patient anxiety, and, almost inevitably, to unnecessary biopsies.

A recent review of more than 1300 prostatectomy cases (performed for prostate cancer) suggests that in our current age of widespread screening (in which the incidence of advanced cancer is low), high PSA levels correlate most closely with large prostate size, but not with the size, stage, or grade of the cancer [62]. A cynic might argue that PSA testing mostly serves to identify old men with big prostates, who incidentally also have a high incidence of prostate cancer. The result has been a five-fold increase in radical prostatectomies, leading to a modest decrease in prostate cancer mortality, but at the cost of tens of thousands of unnecessary prostatectomies [63]. This is basically the problem of "overdetection" or "overdiagnosis;" the likelihood that some of the cancers diagnosed by PSA screening may never become clinically significant. Models using ERSPC data suggest that approximately half of the cancers detected by screening would never have become clinically apparent (i.e., a 50% overdetection rate) [57]. Although we know that overdetection occurs and leads to unnecessary morbidity related to radical treatment (incontinence, impotence, and even operative mortality), the problem remains that in any individual case it is impossible to say whether a screen-detected cancer will or will not ever become clinically relevant.

Given these shortcomings, various methods of improving the performance of the PSA test have been proposed. A lower PSA cutoff would increase sensitivity, but at the inevitable expense of lowering specificity, thereby increasing false-positive results. In an effort to increase specificity, various modifications of PSA testing have been proposed: PSA velocity (the rate of change of PSA over time), PSA density (PSA level compared with prostate volume), and PSA subtypes (free PSA). Lower percentage of free PSA has been associated with a higher risk for cancer, and studies have shown that using the free PSA percentage in men with total PSA 2.6 to 10 ng/mL can eliminate up to 20% of unnecessary biopsies, depending on the cutoffs used [59]. Another strategy that has shown some promise in reducing false-positives involves individualized screening protocols, based on initial PSA level, comorbidities, age, and other risk factors [64,65]. Although these methods may marginally improve the performance of PSA testing, the ultimate solution is to find more accurate and specific biochemical markers for prostate cancer [62].

The current state of PSA screening for prostate cancer is in flux. However, recent epidemiological data strongly suggest that PSA screening has been a factor in the declining mortality from prostate cancer. Studies cited here have only added to concern about false-positives, false-negatives, and overdiagnosis. Current official recommendations reflect this state of uncertainty. In its 2002 update, the United States Preventive Services Task Force changed its rating of PSA screening to a category "I," meaning there is insufficient data to recommend for or against screening [58]. Both the American Cancer Society [66] and the American Urological Association [67] recommend annual screening beginning at age 50 (45 for men at higher risk because of African American heritage or family history of one or more first-degree relatives with prostate cancer). All three organizations recommend that before testing patients should be informed of the uncertain benefits and possible harms related to screening, and that individual preferences and risk factors be taken into account.

Given the present uncertain state of our knowledge and the known inadequacies of the PSA test, the only thing certain is that current recommendations are likely to be refined and changed over the next few years. Schröder sums up our future challenges:

> "It is unlikely that screening in its present form will be acceptable as a health care policy. [An] optimization of the screening tests, limitation of overdiagnosis, a clear definition of the role of comorbidity in decision

making, and greater selectiveness in treatment decisions that take into account the expected individual case history through modeling and aspects of quality of life will have to be considered when future screening strategies are designed" [56].

When to stop screening

A particularly vexing issue that arises in the context of health care of older men is the decision of when to stop screening for cancer. At any age the decision to screen ideally involves a careful balancing of possible benefits against potential harms, but the critical importance of this careful balancing is magnified in the elderly. Although the incidence of most cancers increases with age, actual evidence for benefit of screening in men older than age 70 is limited. The elderly are probably more susceptible to the harms caused by screening, and with advancing age the potential benefit of screening decreases, because competing causes of mortality limit life expectancy. Thus, on theoretical grounds we can say that at *some* age, the potential harms of screening will begin to outweigh the benefits.

Given these concerns, as well as the lack of good data regarding screening for cancer in elderly men, we must rely on general principles when counseling our older patients about screening. A recent position statement from the American Geriatrics Society [68] and a decision model by Walter and Covinsky [69] describe these guiding principles. First, the patient's life expectancy should be considered, taking into account the risk of death from any significant comorbidities. Second, in considering the potential benefit of screening, what is the "lead time" of the test, or how long would it take for an actual benefit to accrue to the patient? Presumably, if the "lead time" exceeds the patient's anticipated life expectancy, screening will have little benefit. The third consideration is the possible harm of screening. What is the potential for anxiety, discomfort, cost, and morbidity that might arise from pursuing positive screening results? Finally and most importantly, all of these should be considered within the context of the individual patient's values and preferences, which implies the need for a careful discussion of these issues with each patient or his caregivers.

For colorectal cancer screening, there is some information that it takes at least 5 years to see a mortality benefit from screening, so presumably there is little value in screening when life expectancy is less than this. Screening studies have generally been restricted to patients younger than age 80, so any benefit to those beyond that age is unproven [31]. A critical unknown is whether previous negative screening should be taken into account: it is quite possible that a man with a normal screening colonoscopy at age 70 is at very low risk for ever having colon cancer.

In the case of prostate cancer screening, major guidelines agree that men who have less than a 10-year life expectancy or who are older than age 70 to

75 are unlikely to benefit from screening [58,66,67]. Despite these guidelines it appears that many older American men are receiving prostate cancer screening from which they are unlikely to benefit. Data from a 2001 nationwide survey show that men in the 70- to 79-year age group have a higher prevalence of PSA testing within the past year (69%) than any other age group. Even in those 80 and older, 56% of men have had PSA testing within the past year [70].

Summary

Screening for cancer, with the promise of early detection and improved outcomes, is an accepted and intuitively appealing part of primary care medicine. However, because potential biases can inflate the apparent benefit of screening tests, RCTs with mortality as an endpoint are the only way to prove unequivocally that screening benefits patients. Of the common cancers affecting men, only screening for colorectal cancer meets this high standard. Screening for lung cancer with computed tomography can detect cancer at an earlier stage, but as yet there is no proof that this results in improved outcomes. Screening for prostate cancer with PSA testing appears to have favorably altered the epidemiology of that disease, with fewer men presenting with late stage disease and a 20% decline in mortality over the past 15 years, but overdiagnosis, false-positives, and false-negatives appear to be relatively common problems.

References

[1] Woodwell DA, Cherry DK. National Ambulatory Medical Care Survey: 2002 summary. Advance data from Vital and Health Statistics. No. 346 (Aug 26, 2004). CDC. Available at: http://www.cdc.gov/nchs/data/ad/ad346.pdf. Accessed November 23, 2004.

[2] Gates TJ. Concepts and controversies in cancer screening. Am J Cancer 2003;2:395–402.

[3] US Preventive Services Task Force. Screening for cervical cancer. Guide to clinical preventive services. 2nd edition. Baltimore(MD): Williams & Wilkins; 1996, p. 105–17.

[4] Schwartz LM, Woloshin S, Fowler FJ, et al. Enthusiasm for cancer screening in the US. JAMA 2004;291:71–8.

[5] Collins MM, Barry MJ. Controversies in prostate cancer screening: analogies to the early lung cancer screening debate. JAMA 1996;276:1976–9.

[6] Wallace RB. Screening for early and asymptomatic conditions. In: Wallace RB, editor. Public Health and Preventative Medicine. 14th edition. Norwalk (CT): Appleton & Lange; 1998. p. 907–8.

[7] Gates TJ. Screening for cancer: evaluating the evidence. Am Fam Phy 2001;63:513–22.

[8] Marshall KG. The ethics of informed consent for preventive screening programs. Can Med Assoc J 1996;155:377–82.

[9] Sackett DL, Haynes RB, Guyatt GH, et al. Clinical epidemiology: a basic science for clinical medicine. 2nd edition. Boston: Little, Brown, and Company; 1991. p. 153–70.

[10] Malm HM. Medical screening and the value of early detection: when unwarranted faith leads to unethical recommendations. Hastings Cent Rep 1999;29:26–37.

[11] Doukas DJ, Fetters M, Ruffin MT, et al. Ethical considerations in the provision of controversial screening tests. Arch Fam Med 1997;6:486–90.

[12] Black WC. Overdiagnosis: an underrecognized cause of confusion and harm in cancer screening. J Natl Cancer Inst 2000;92:1280–2.
[13] Frame PS, Carlson SJ. A critical review of periodic health screening using specific screening criteria. J Fam Pract 1975;2:29–35.
[14] Canadian Task Force on the periodic health examination. The periodic health examination. Can Med Assoc J 1979;121:1194–254.
[15] US Preventive Services Task Force. Guide to clinical preventive services. Washington, DC: US Department of Health & Human Services; 1989.
[16] Black WC, Haggstrom DA, Welch HG. All-cause mortality in randomized trials of cancer screening. J Natl Cancer Inst 2002;94:167–73.
[17] Taber L, Duffy SW, Yen M, et al. All-cause mortality among breast cancer patients in a screening trial: support for breast cancer mortality as an end point. J Med Screen 2002; 9:159–62.
[18] Juffs HG, Tannock IF. Screening trials are even more difficult than we thought they were. J Natl Cancer Inst 2002;94:156–7.
[19] Marshall KG. Influence of reporting methods on perception of benefits. Can Med Assoc J 1996;154:493–9.
[20] Cook RJ, Sackett DL. The number needed to treat: a clinically useful measure of treatment effect. BMJ 1995;310:452–4.
[21] Rembold CM. Number needed to screen: development of a statistic for disease screening. BMJ 1998;317:307–12.
[22] Jemal A, Murray T, Ward E, et al. Cancer statistics 2005. CA Cancer J Clin 2005;55:10–30.
[23] Screening for testicular cancer: a brief evidence update for the USPSTF. AHRQ Pub. No. 05–0553-B, February 2004.
[24] Canadian Task Force on preventive health care. CTFPHC systematic reviews and recommendation. Available at: http://www.ctfphc.org. Accessed January 10, 2005.
[25] Zoorob R, Anderson R, Cefalu C, et al. Cancer screening guidelines. Am Fam Phy 2001;63: 1101–12.
[26] Towler BP, Irwig L, Glasziou P, et al. Screening for colorectal cancer using the fecal occult blood test, hemoccult. Cochrane Database Syst Rev 2000;2:CD001216.
[27] Fletcher RH. Review: fecal occult blood test screening reduces colorectal cancer mortality. ACP J Club 1999;130:13.
[28] Sonnenberg A, Delco F, Inadomi JM. Cost-effectiveness of colonoscopy in screening for colorectal cancer. Ann Intern Med 2000;133:573–84.
[29] Frazier AL, Colditz GA, Fuchs CS, et al. Cost-effectiveness of screening for colorectal cancer in the general population. JAMA 2000;284:1954–61.
[30] Lieberman DA, Weiss DG. One-time screening for colorectal cancer with combined fecal occult-blood testing and examination of the distal colon. N Engl J Med 2001;345: 555–60.
[31] US Preventive Services Task Force. Screening for colorectal cancer: recommendations and rationale. Ann Intern Med 2002;137:129–31.
[32] Smith RA, Cokkinides V, Eyre HJ. American Cancer Society guidelines for the early detection of cancer 2005. CA Cancer J Clin 2005;55:31–44.
[33] Pickhardt PJ, Choi JR, Hwang I, et al. Computed tomographic virtual colonoscopy to screen for colorectal neoplasia in asymptomatic adults. N Engl J Med 2003;349:2191–200.
[34] Cotton PB, Durkalski VL, Pineau BC, et al. Computed tomographic colonography (virtual colonoscopy). A multicenter comparison with standard colonoscopy for detection of colorectal neoplasia. JAMA 2004;291:1713–9.
[35] Wender RC. Barriers to screening for colorectal cancer screening. Gastrointest Endosc Clin N Am 2002;12:145–70.
[36] Hardcastle JD, Chamberlain JD, Robinson M, et al. Randomized controlled trial of fecal-occult blood screening for colorectal cancer. Lancet 1996;348:1472–7.

[37] Tazi MA, Faivre J, Dassonville F, et al. Participation in fecal occult blood screening for colorectal cancer in a well defined French population: results of five screening rounds from 1988 to 1996. J Med Screen 1997;4:147–51.
[38] Ruffin MT, Gorenflo DW, Woodman B. Predictors of screening for breast, cervical, colorectal, and prostatic cancer among community-based primary care practices. J Am Board Fam Pract 2000;13:1–10.
[39] Brawarsky P, Brooks DR, Mucci LA. Correlates of colorectal cancer testing in Massachusetts men and women. Prev Med 2003;36:659–68.
[40] Donovan JM, Syngal S. Colorectal cancer in women: an underappreciated but preventable risk. J Womens Health 1998;7:45–8.
[41] Manser RL, Irving LB, Stone C, et al. Screening for lung cancer. Cochrane Database Syst Rev. 2001;3:CD001991. Review. Update in Cochrane Database Syst Rev. 2004;(1): CD001991.
[42] Patz EF, Goodman PC, Bepler G. Screening for lung cancer. N Engl J Med 2000;343: 1627–33.
[43] Henschke CI, McCauley DI, Yankelevitz DF, et al. Early lung cancer action project: overall design and findings from baseline screening. Lancet 1999;354:99–105.
[44] Swenson SJ, Jett JR, Hartman TE, et al. Lung cancer screening with CT: Mayo clinic experience. Radiology 2003;226:756–61.
[45] Henschke C, Shusuke S, Markowitz S, et al. International early lung cancer action project (I-ELCAP): evaluation of low-dose CT screening. Abstract presented at the Radiological Society of North America. Chicago, November 28, 2004.
[46] Humphrey LL, Teutsch S, Johnson M. Lung cancer screening with sputum cytologic examination, chest radiography and computed tomography: an update for the US Preventive Services Task Force. Ann Intern Med 2004;140:740–53.
[47] Grannis FW. Lung cancer overdiagnosis bias. [editorial] Chest 2001;119:322–3.
[48] Jett JR. Spiral computed tomography screening for lung cancer is ready for prime time. Am J Respir Crit Care Med 2001;163:812–3.
[49] US Preventive Services Task Force. Lung cancer screening: recommendation statement. Ann Intern Med 2004;140:738–9.
[50] Bach PB, Niewoehner DE, Black WC. Screening for lung cancer: the guidelines. Chest 2003; 123:835–85.
[51] Aberle DR, Gamsu G, Henschke CI, et al. A consensus statement of the Society of Thoracic Radiology: screening for lung cancer with helical computed tomography. J Thoracic Imaging 2001;16:65–8.
[52] Merenstein D. Winners and losers. JAMA 2004;292:15–6.
[53] Oottamasathien S, Crawford ED. Should routine screening for prostate-specific antigen be recommended? Arch Intern Med 2003;163:661–2.
[54] Crawford ED. Epidemiology of prostate cancer. Urology 2003;62(Suppl 6A):3–12.
[55] Wilson SS, Crawford ED. Screening for prostate cancer: current recommendations. Urol Clin N Am 2004;31:219–26.
[56] Schröder FH. Screening for prostate cancer. Urol Clin North Am 2003;30:239–51.
[57] Otto SJ, de Koning HJ. Update on screening and early detection of prostate cancer. Curr Opin Urol 2004;14:151–6.
[58] US Preventive Services Task Force. Screening for prostate cancer: recommendations and rationale. Ann Intern Med 2002;137:915–6.
[59] Han M, Gann PH, Catalona WJ. Prostate-specific antigen and screening for prostate cancer. Med Clin North Am 2004;88:245–65.
[60] Frankel S, Smith GD, Donovan J, et al. Screening for prostate cancer. Lancet 2003;361: 1122–8.
[61] Thompson IM, Pauler DK, Goodman PJ, et al. Prevalence of prostate cancer among men with a prostate-specific antigen level $\leq$ 4.0 ng per milliliter. N Engl J Med 2004;350:2239–46.

[62] Stamey TA, Caldwell M, McNeal JE, et al. The prostate specific antigen era in the United States is over for prostate cancer: What happened in the last 20 years? J Urol 2004;172: 1297–301.

[63] Stephenson RA. Prostate cancer trends in the era of prostate-specific antigen: an update of incidence, mortality, and clinical factors from the SEER database. Urol Clin North Am 2002;29:173–81.

[64] Antenor JV, Han M, Roehl KA, et al. Relationship between initial prostate specific antigen level and subsequent prostate cancer detection in a longitudinal screening study. J Urol 2004; 172:90–3.

[65] Finne P, Finne R, Bangma C, et al. Algorithms based on prostate-specific antigen (PSA), free PSA, digital rectal examination and prostate volume reduce false-positive PSA results in prostate cancer screening. Int J Cancer 2004;111:310–5.

[66] American Cancer Society. ACS cancer detection guidelines: prostate cancer. Available at: http://www.cancer.org/docroot/PED/content/PED_2_3X_ACS_Cancer_Detection_Guidelines. Accessed January 25, 2005.

[67] American Urological Association PSA Best Practice Policy Task Force. Prostate-specific antigen (PSA) best practice policy. Oncology 2000;14:267–86.

[68] American Geriatrics Society Ethics Committee. Health screening decisions for older adults: The AGS position paper. J Am Geriatr Soc 2003;51:270–1.

[69] Walter LC, Covinsky KE. Cancer screening in elderly patients: A framework for individualized decision making. JAMA 2001;285:2750–6.

[70] Sirovich BE, Schwartz LM, Woloshin S. Screening men for prostate and colorectal cancer in the Unites States: Does practice reflect the evidence? JAMA 2003;289:1414–20.

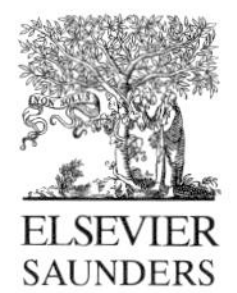

ELSEVIER
SAUNDERS

Nurs Clin N Am 43 (2008) 307–322

NURSING
CLINICS
OF NORTH AMERICA

The Older Cancer Patient

Heidi K. White, MD, MHS[a,b,*],
Harvey J. Cohen, MD[a,b,c]

[a]*Geriatrics Division, Duke University School of Medicine, 3502 Bluezone, Box 3003, Durham, NC 27710, USA*

[b]*Geriatric Research, Education, and Clinical Center, Veterans Affairs Medical Center, 508 Fulton Street, Durham, NC 27705, USA*

[c]*Center for the Study of Aging and Human Development, Geriatrics Division, Duke University Medical Center, Box 3003, Durham, NC 27710, USA*

Cancer is a common problem in the older adult population and the second leading cause of death for both men and women. More than half of cancers occur in adults over the age of 65 years. The biologic, psychologic, and social aspects of the aging process must be considered for optimal screening, diagnosis, and treatment to occur in this population. The growing number of older adults facing a cancer diagnosis in conjunction with other acute and chronic conditions makes it imperative for primary care physicians, geriatricians, oncologists, surgeons, radiation oncologists, and virtually all specialists to consider the merits of geriatric assessment and treatment for optimal management. Of course cancer is not one disease but many. Rather than address even a short list of common cancers, this article focuses on aspects of the aging process that impact cancer development, progression, and treatment, along with principles that can be applied to the care of older patients who have cancer.

Principles of aging in the care of older adult patients who have cancer

Understanding what makes the older adult patient who has cancer different from the middle-aged patient who has cancer, apart from comorbid illness, which can be a burden in both groups, is an important place to start conceptualizing appropriate care for this group of individuals (Table 1).

A version of this article was previously published in the September 2006 issue of the Medical Clinics of North America.

* Corresponding author. Geriatrics Division, Duke University School of Medicine, 3502 Bluezone, Box 3003, Durham, NC 27710.

E-mail address: white031@mc.duke.edu (H.K. White).

0029-6465/08/$ - see front matter
doi:10.1016/j.cnur.2008.03.003

Table 1
Selected aspects of aging and their impact on older adults who have cancer

Aging process	Impact on older adult patient who has cancer
Decreasing homeostatic reserve	• Decreased ability to tolerate cancer treatment without adverse events or complications • Assessment is needed to measure functional reserves (eg, creatinine clearance, cognitive screening)
Heterogeneity	• Assessment parameters other than chronologic age will best characterize an individual patient's ability to undergo cancer-specific treatment with acceptable levels of toxicity, and quality of life (eg, comorbidities, functional status) • A particular patient may exhibit adequate reserves in some organ system and more limited reserves in others
Declining adaptability	• Prolonged recovery and rehabilitation • Increased sensitivity to drug effects
Altered pharmacokinetics	• Potential for poor drug absorption, higher peak concentrations, and prolonged half-life because of altered excretion
Altered pharmacodynamics	• Increased sensitivity to toxicity of drugs (eg, higher rates of neutropenia, higher rates of mucositis)

Decreasing homeostatic reserve

Aging results in a steady decline in physiologic reserve capacity in most organ systems and dysregulation in others. These changes are related to the passage of time and are not the result of disease processes but do increase the vulnerability to disease. These changes generally are imperceptible at rest or in the individual's steady state but become apparent under stress of the system. Important changes that result in decreased reserve capacity include impaired glucose tolerance, decreased FEV_1 and FVC, decreased creatinine clearance and glomerular filtration rate, decreased muscle mass (sarcopenia), decreased bone mass, decreased brain blood flow and impaired autoregulation of blood flow, decreased dark adaptation of vision, decreased odor detection, and loss of high-frequency auditory tones, to name only a few. An example of decreased bone marrow reserve is evident in higher rates of neutropenia among older patients treated with full-dose chemotherapeutic regimens for non-Hodgkin lymphoma [1]. As aging advances the loss of reserve capacity progresses and becomes evident even in a steady state; this advanced stage of absent reserves and dysregulation is being defined as the syndrome of frailty.

Heterogeneity in aging

Despite these predictable age-related changes that decrease reserve capacity and increase the vulnerability of older adults to progressively smaller and smaller stresses, there is an amazing degree of heterogeneity that is evident in the aging population. This heterogeneity is most evident when comparing older adults to one another but it is also evident in the variability of age-related changes within organ systems of a given individual. For example, in the Baltimore Longitudinal study glomerular filtration rate on average declined 1 mL/min/y. But as many as 30% of individuals experienced no decline, whereas others experienced a decline of up to 2 mL/min/y [2]. In addition to presumed genetic differences that influence aging rates, behavioral factors, such as diet and exercise, play an important role.

Slowing of the adaptive response

Older adults adapt more slowly to environmental stressors. Aging has been defined as a progressive loss of adaptability of an individual organism as time passes. This loss is compellingly demonstrated in the marathon records by age group published by the US Corporate Athletic Association [3]. By this listing men aged 30 to 34 currently hold the best time of 2:19:04; however, the record for men aged 65 to 99 is 3:26:38, more than an hour longer. Although it is great news that men of this age are capable of completing marathons at a pace that would outdo many younger marathon runners, clearly older men do not possess the same degree of adaptability in this sport. In a perhaps more immediately relevant example, a slower (less vigorous) adaptive response may explain in part the increased susceptibility with age of normal tissues to chemotherapy. Mucosa, hemopoietic cells, the heart, and the nervous system are more susceptible to chemotherapy. For example, in patients who have cancer of the colon age is an independent risk factor for the development of mucositis induced by fluorinated pyrimidines [4].

Alterations in pharmacokinetics and pharmacodynamics of antineoplastic therapy

Aging has a profound impact on the pharmacokinetics and pharmacodynamics of antineoplastic therapy [5]. Pharmacokinetics is what the body does to the drug in terms of absorption, distribution, metabolism, and excretion. With increasing age absorption may be reduced by decreased gastrointestinal motility, decreased secretion of gastric enzymes, and mucosal atrophy. Drug distribution is a function of body composition and the concentration of plasma proteins. In older adults body fat increases and water content decreases; this translates into a larger volume of distribution for fat-soluble drugs and reduced volume of distribution for water-soluble drugs, which lead to changes in peak concentration and alterations in half-life. Metabolism mainly occurs in the liver and is not affected strongly by aging processes but can be altered by surgical stress and illness [6,7]. Excretion is most affected by the gradual decline in glomerular filtration rate.

Pharmacodynamics refers to what the drug does to the body, primarily referring to alterations in sensitivity that may lead to adverse events. For example, the plasma concentration of midazolam at which 50% of patients will be nonresponsive to the stimulus of verbal command decreases steadily with patient age [8]. It is more difficult to study pharmacodynamics because of the confounding effects of pharmacokinetics, which may appear to increase sensitivity when in actuality drug levels are elevated above typical levels because of alterations in distribution, metabolism, or excretion.

The geriatrics adage, "start low, go slow," means start with a low dosage and advance the dosage slowly. This simple yet effective approach has become a mainstay for avoiding problems because of altered pharmacokinetics and pharmacodynamics. It may not be as applicable for cancer-specific treatment as it is for symptom-specific treatment, however, because lower dosages of chemotherapy may rob older adults of the benefits of desired treatment effects while minimizing toxicity.

Aging biology in the development of cancer

The biologic basis of cancer development is multidimensional. Disruption of genetic integrity is a cornerstone of this process. Alterations in the cellular environment also are important. These factors lead to the multistep process of cellular changes that result in neoplasia. The relationship between cancer biology and aging biology is beginning to unfold. The general increase in frequency of cancer with age makes the relationship between aging and cancer biology somewhat intuitive, but not all cancers increase in incidence with age. The incidence of breast, colon, and prostate cancers increase with age, whereas cervical cancer does not. The influence of aging on cancer biology remains uncertain. Some cancers appear more aggressive in advanced age, such as acute myelogenous leukemia, Hodgkin disease, and non-Hodgkin lymphoma, whereas other cancers, such as breast and prostate cancer, may become more indolent with advanced age. The linkage between aging and cancer biology may differ by cancer type and is influenced by environmental exposures and lifestyle choices. At a basic level aging provides the necessary time for chemical mutagens, radiation, and free radicals to promote genetic damage and aged cells may be more susceptible to these carcinogens. Cellular senescence is an important link between aging and cancer. This theory holds that nonmalignant cells have a finite replicative potential that is governed largely by telomere shortening. Telomeres, specialized regions of reiterative DNA at the ends of chromosomes, gradually shorten with successive replicative cycles. This shortening leads to the accumulation of senescent cells with age. Malignant cells overcome telomere shortening by upregulating production of telomerase [9]. Research regarding this linkage between aging and cancer is quickly accelerating our understanding of the interplay between cancer biology and aging biology, but other linkages are coming to light also, such as decreased ability to repair DNA, oncogene activation or amplification, decreased tumor suppressor gene activity, microenvironment alterations, and decreased immune surveillance [10].

Comprehensive geriatric assessment for patients who have cancer

Because chronologic age is not an adequate indicator of response to cancer treatment and tolerance of toxicity, other factors need to be identified that characterize a "functional age," assist in developing the most appropriate treatment plan, and further our understanding of what factors do influence outcomes. In the last 10 years there has been a growing recognition of the potential for comprehensive geriatric assessment (CGA) to improve the care of older adults who have cancer [11]. The International Society of Geriatric Oncology recommends the use of CGA in the evaluation of older patients who have cancer to detect unaddressed problems and improve functional status and, possibly, survival [12]. Components of the geriatric assessment are outlined in Table 2 along with screening tools, examples of detailed test components, and additional resources. CGA is "a multi disciplinary evaluation in which the multiple problems of older adults are uncovered, described, and explained, if possible, and in which the resources and strengths of the person are catalogued, need for services assessed, and a coordinated care plan developed to focus interventions on the person's problems" [13].

Geriatric assessment has been studied in various settings that include specialized hospital units, hospital consultation services alone or with outpatient followup, clinic-based services, and in-home assessments. CGA has been shown to have positive effects on various health outcomes, such as prevention of disability progression, reduction of fall risk, rates of hospitalization, and nursing home admission. CGA is most effective when programs have control over implementation of recommendations and extended followup. Meta-analyses have suggested an impact on mortality [14,15], but more recent multi-institutional randomized controlled trials show no impact on mortality [16,17]. The results of studies of cost-effectiveness have been varied but generally favorable [17,18].

Specific trials of geriatric assessment outcomes in the oncologic setting are lacking. Some studies have suggested promise for the approach, however. One study using hospital inpatient geriatric care units for older adults who have cancer has shown improvements in psychologic status and pain management compared with usual care [19]. Another approach that has been implemented successfully has been to use primarily self-report components [20,21]. A pilot study of CGA by Extermann and colleagues in older women with breast cancer identified multiple undiagnosed problems [22]. Several studies indicate that when important predictors of mortality, such as cancer stage at diagnosis and age, are controlled, the burden of comorbid illness is an important predictor of mortality [23,24]. Specific comorbidities,

Table 2
Comprehensive geriatric assessment

Dimension	Screen	Detailed assessment	Resources
Medical			
Nutrition	Height, weight, serum albumin, cholesterol	BMI, Mini Nutritional Assessment	Dietician, speech therapist
Vision	"Describe any visual limitations."	Snellen Eye Chart	Ophthalmologist, optometrist
Hearing	"Do you have any trouble with your hearing?" Finger rub test	Audioscope	Audiologist
Mobility/balance	Observed standing up, ambulation, and sitting down	Timed Get Up and Go [58], measured gait speed	Physical therapist, medically supervised exercise programs
Urinary incontinence	Screening questions	Urodynamic testing, urinalysis and urine culture	Urologist, gynecologist, geriatrician
Comorbidities	Review of systems, medical record	Activity, severity, stability	Primary care physician, specialists
Medications	Review medication by having the patient bring all medication bottles to the visit	Ask patient to explain regimen, reason for each drug, and potential adverse effects	PharmacistPrimary care physician
Cognitive	"Do you have any memory or thinking problems?" Get permission to ask the same question of family members, Minicog	Mini Mental Status Exam	Neuropsychological testing, referral to geriatrician, psychiatrist, neurologist
Affective	Clinical observation, "Do you often feel sad or blue?"	Geriatric Depression Scale Koenig Depression Screen	Psychiatrist, psychologist, social worker

Functional status	ADL Do you need help using the bathroom, bathing, dressing eating? IADL "Can you use the telephone, pay your bills, shop, drive a car?"	Katz ADL and IADL scale	Physical therapist, occupational therapist, speech therapist
Social support	"Who would help you in an emergency?"	Detailed assessment of caregiver involvement and extended social support	Social worker, home health services, hospice
Economic	"Do you have the financial resources to meet your current and future needs?"	Health insurance Drug coverage	Social worker
Environment	Home safety checklist	Home visit	Occupational therapist, physical therapist, home health nurse
Advance directives	"Do you have an advanced directive?"	Detailed discussion	Social worker

Abbreviations: ADL, activities of daily living; BMI, body mass index; IADL, instrumental activities of daily living.

Data from Balducci L, Extermann M. Management of cancer in the older person: a practical approach. Oncologist 2000;5:224–37 and Reuben DB. Geriatric assessment in oncology. Cancer 1997;80:1311–6.

especially depression and cognitive impairment, are under-recognized in the oncology setting [25,26]. Comorbidity and functional status are independent predictors in older adult patients who have cancer and both need to be assessed [27]. Traditional oncologic measures of function, such as Karnofsky and Eastern Cooperative Oncology Group, are incomplete predictors in the elderly [27,28]. Ultimately, CGA should evaluate not only comorbidities and functional status but also stages or states of aging along with functional and coping (psychosocial) reserves that accurately predict therapeutic outcomes and improve outcomes through tailored treatment strategies.

In this vein CGA may be used to recognize frailty, a developing concept of a phenotype that is strongly predictive of falls, disability, hospitalization, and mortality [29]. This phenotype is not synonymous with comorbidity or disability. Comorbidity is likely causative and disability should be considered an outcome. Frailty is attributable to underlying processes of aging and may be particularly useful in uncovering limited or absent reserve capacity associated with advanced aging. Recognizing older adults who appear stable and functional but have limited ability to recover from the stressors associated with cancer treatment may be extremely helpful in tailoring treatment plans [30]. At present there are competing definitions of frailty. Balducci and colleagues define frailty as one or more of the following: dependence in at least one activity of daily living (ADL), three or more serious comorbid conditions, and one or more geriatric syndromes [31]. Fried and colleagues define frailty by the presence of three of the following criteria: involuntary weight loss $\geq 10\%$ of body weight over 1 year, fatigue, weakness (grip strength), slow walking speed, and low physical activity [29].

To date it seems that few specialists caring for older patients who have cancer use CGA on a regular basis, despite a general acknowledgment that age alone is not an adequate means of making treatment decisions [32,33]. This lack of assessment may be in large part because of a perceived impracticality of adopting a potentially time-consuming procedure with still unclear benefits for patient care. Cancer specialists are beginning to do the hard work of determining how to make CGA practical in usual care settings, however. There are several potential answers to this dilemma. Using primarily self-report components may optimize data gathering while minimizing staff time, but this may be less practical for more impaired individuals or diverse patient populations with limited literacy or English proficiency. Using hospital inpatient geriatric care units for older adults who have cancer may be a viable option in locations where these are available. In academic settings cancer specialists may be able to work in conjunction with geriatricians to manage more complicated older adult patients who have cancer. Also, cancer specialists should consider partnering with other clinical professionals in the implementation of CGA. Nurses, social workers, and midlevel practitioners can and should be part of the geriatric assessment process. A team approach to care has already been implemented to bring together the various cancer specialists to ensure that treatment modalities, including chemotherapy, radiation, and surgery, are implemented seamlessly; such programs can incorporate geriatric assessment into this team management framework. Screening tools may be another way of limiting time commitments, reserving full-blown CGA to those most likely to benefit from it. Screening tools may be informal, such as the screening questions outlined in Table 2. Alternatively, the Vulnerable Elders Survey 13 (VES-13) represents a formal means of predicting functional decline and death that also may be a viable screening tool (Fig. 1) [34]. The incorporation of CGA into clinical trials is of critical importance if we are to better delineate which patients with functional and cognitive limitations are appropriate for specific treatment regimens. This methodology will allow for comparison of patient characteristics across studies.

Tailoring treatment

CGA also can facilitate the process of tailoring treatment for individual patients (Table 3). The information collected should be used to establish goals of care; direct cancer-specific and symptom-specific treatment in light of comorbidities, functional status, psychological and social resources; and begin or review advanced planning (eg, living will, health care power of attorney, use of feeding tube).

Cancer-specific treatment

When carefully selected, older adult patients who have cancer undergoing the range of cancer treatment modalities experience similar responses to those seen in younger patients. Surgeons have been able to select carefully older adults who successfully undergo curative and palliative surgical procedures. Careful preoperative assessment, management of comorbidities, appropriate anesthesia management, and meticulous postoperative care have produced outcomes similar to those experienced by younger patients [35]. Radiation therapy is successful in older adults who have cancer and has developed its technical specificity for curative and palliative application with improved tolerability for older adults. Hormonal therapy is effective in older adult patients who have cancer of the breast, uterus, and prostate. With the advent of effective supportive therapy for the toxicity associated with chemotherapy more physicians have been willing to extend this treatment option to older patients, even those with some functional limitations and comorbidities. Growth factors, such as granulocyte colony-stimulating factor, modify or eliminate immunosuppressant effects. Cytoprotective agents, such as dexrazoxane, modify the cardiotoxic effects of doxorubicin. Newer antiemetics and improved techniques of chemotherapy administration also have opened the door of effective treatment to a wider range of older adult patients who have cancer. Important studies, such as the recent study of

VES-13

1. **Age** ______________________

SCORE: *1 POINT FOR AGE 75-84*
3 POINT FOR AGE ≥ 85

2. **In general, compared to other people you age, would you say that your health is:**

- ☐ **Poor,*** *(1 POINT)*
- ☐ **Fair,*** *(1 POINT)*
- ☐ **Good.**
- ☐ **Very good, or**
- ☐ **Excellent**

SCORE: *1 POINT FOR FAIR or POOR*

3. **How difficulty, on average, do you have with the following physical activities:**

	No Difficulty	A little Difficulty	Some Difficulty	A Lot of Difficulty	Unable to do
a. stooping, crouching or kneeling?	☐	☐	☐	☐*	☐*
b. lifting, or carrying objects as heavy as 10 pounds?	☐	☐	☐	☐*	☐*
c. reaching or extending arms above shoulder level?	☐	☐	☐	☐*	☐*
d. writing, or handling and grasping small objects?	☐	☐	☐	☐*	☐*
e. walking a quarter of a mile?	☐	☐	☐	☐*	☐*
f. heavy housework such as scrubbing floors or washing windows?	☐	☐	☐	☐*	☐*

SCORE: 1 POINT FOR EACH RESPONSE IN Q3a THROUGH f. MAXIMUM OF 2 POINTS.*

4. **Because of your health or a physical condition, do you have any difficulty:**

   a. **shopping for personal items (like toilet items or medicined)?**

   ☐ **YES → Do you get help with shopping?** ☐ **YES *** ☐ **NO**
   ☐ **NO**
   ☐ **DON'T DO → is that because of your health?** ☐ **YES *** ☐ **NO**

   b. **managing money (like keeping track of expenses or paying bills)?**

   ☐ **YES → Do you get help with managing money?** ☐ **YES *** ☐ **NO**

Fig. 1. Vulnerable Elders Survey. A score of 4 or more is associated with a four times greater risk for death or functional decline over 2 years among community-dwelling elders. (*Adapted from* Saliba D, Elliott M, Rubenstein LZ, et al. The Vulnerable Elders Survey: a tool for identifying vulnerable older people in the community. J Amer Geriatr Soc 2001;49(12):1691–9; with permission.)

adjuvant chemotherapy for lymph node–positive breast cancer, are confirming that older adults are just as likely to benefit from chemotherapy as younger adults [36].

It is important that older adults are allowed to make treatment decisions with explanations of all reasonable treatment options, including forgoing cancer-specific treatment. To make fully informed decisions they need

Table 3
CGA-based cancer treatment plan

Treatment type	Components
Cancer-specific treatment	Surgery
	Chemotherapy
	Hormonal therapy
	Radiation therapy
Symptom-specific therapy	Example: pain relief
	Medication, exercise, heat/cold, alternative therapies (eg, acupuncture), relaxation techniques, nerve blocks
Supportive therapy	Dietary support
	Exercise prescription
	Support groups
End-of-life care	Address advance directives
	Periodically review goals of care

information regarding likely outcomes, adverse effects, and a description of the usual experience of treatment participation (frequency and length of procedures, usual recovery period, and so forth). If the treating physician is aware of functional limitations, cognitive impairment, or limitations of social support through the process of CGA, this allows for a more productive discussion of treatment options with the ability to anticipate and plan for how these issues may impact the treatment process and outcomes. For example, older adults who have cognitive impairment are at increased risk for developing delirium during hospitalization. Recognizing this potential complication can allow for interventions, such as family members staying with the patient around the clock, to be anticipated and planned. Many older adults rely heavily on close family members to assist them in treatment decisions. The physician can facilitate this process by inviting and encouraging the patient to bring family members to appointments.

Treatment goals should be established clearly between the physician and patient. These goals should be reassessed periodically depending on factors that may precipitate change, such as a lack of response to therapy or a significant change in functional status. Communication helps to ensures that the goals of care are reflected in the course of treatment [37].

Symptom-specific treatment

Whether or not patients decide to undergo cancer-specific treatment, symptom-specific treatment should be part of the treatment plan from diagnosis until death. Cancer specialists are becoming more and more adept at recognizing and treating cancer-related and treatment-related symptoms [38]. For example, fatigue is a particularly common symptom, especially in advanced stages of cancer. Treatment modalities include education, exercise, treatment of anemia, antidepressants, and psychostimulants.

Pain is a common symptom experienced from early to late stages of cancer. Pain should be systematically assessed. Options include a visual descriptor scale containing a set of numbers with words representing different levels of pain. A visual analog scale typically uses a 10-cm line marked "no pain" on the left and "worst possible pain" on the right. The pain thermometer is a visual scale that allows patients to place their pain on a vertical scale that resembles a thermometer. The Faces pain scale provides a series of faces depicting various degrees of facial grimacing. Perhaps most frequently, patients are asked without a visual device such as those just described to rate their pain on a scale of 0 to 10, with 0 being no pain and 10 being the worst possible pain. The American Geriatrics Society guidelines for persistent pain management are helpful in developing a comprehensive treatment plan that is based on anticipatory treatment of pain with scheduled dosing rather than dosing as needed. This topic is addressed thoroughly elsewhere in this volume.

Depression is fairly common among older adults who have chronic illness. Rates in patients who have cancer have been estimated at 17% to 33% [39,40]. Women who have severe illness, poor functional status, and advanced cancer are most at risk [40,41]. Multiple validated screening tools are available and should be used routinely, given the high prevalence of depression among patients who have cancer [42–44]. Treatment options include antidepressants, counseling, and electroconvulsive therapy.

Supportive care

Efforts currently are underway to assess the impact of diet and exercise prescriptions on the trajectory of functional decline and quality of life in newly diagnosed older adult patients who have cancer. Such efforts signal an acknowledgment of the motivation among patients who have cancer to make lifestyle changes and the potential for supportive interventions in addition to cancer-specific and symptom-specific treatments to improve the functional status and quality of life [45,46]. In another study, older patients who had cancer who also had mouth or tooth problems making it hard for them to eat experienced lower quality of life, poor emotional health, lower levels of physical functioning, and greater pain than patients without these problems [47]. This study emphasizes the impact that comorbid conditions can have on patients who have cancer, especially if they are not optimally identified and treated. In addition to comprehensive medical care, psychosocial interventions for the patient and caregiver can be extremely important. Supportive care needs to continue long term for cancer survivors who report a greater degree of disability than their counterparts without a history of cancer [48].

Psychosocial support is extremely important for the patient who has cancer, because the psychosocial demands of the illness course make an independent contribution to survival outcomes [49]. Support also should be available for the caregiver, because despite the many benefits of caregiving, such as greater intimacy, satisfaction, and gaining meaning and purpose in life, there are also substantial mental, physical, social, and economic costs [50].

End-of-life care

End-of-life care should begin as early as possible in the course of a life-threatening illness. An important initial step is asking about advanced directives, such as living will and health care power of attorney. If patients are unfamiliar with such documents, their usefulness should be explained and written information provided. It is important for patients to understand that choosing a less aggressive treatment plan does not mean they will forgo the involvement of a physician. The phrase "nothing more can be done" should not be used; physicians need to convey a willingness to stay involved with care and symptom management up until the moment of death [51]. Ideally the patient's goals should be elicited at every stage of treatment and should be reflected in the course of treatment that is provided [37]. End-of-life care is thoroughly covered elsewhere in this volume.

The emergence of geriatric oncology

Although 61% of new cases of cancer occur among the elderly they represent only 32% of participants in phase II and III clinical trials [52]. When comorbidities are controlled, age remains a strong predictor of whether or not a patient who has cancer will be offered a clinical trial, but when offered older adults respond with willingness to participate at similar rates [53]. Physicians may have good reasons for not offering clinical trials to older adults, such as protocol requirements that are onerous and not easily appreciated on enrollment, treatment-specific issues, including toxicity, and older patients' medical and cognitive characteristics that may not exclude them but will hinder compliance with study requirements [54]. Insufficient enrollment of older adults in clinical trials is only one example of the inadequacies of current research to meet the needs of this growing population of patients who have cancer. There is an urgent need for further research at the interface of aging and cancer [55]. The lack of sufficient research makes it difficult to answer many of the questions that arise about cancer in older adults. Geriatric oncology represents a viable means of meeting the clinical and research needs of older adults who have cancer [56]. With the help of the John A. Hartford Foundation, gero-oncology training programs have been initiated and leaders are beginning to call for a new subspecialty of gero-oncology. Given the magnitude of the issue of appropriately caring for a growing number of older adults who have cancer, this seems to be a prudent course to pursue [57].

Summary

Providing effective and tolerable cancer treatment for the growing number of older adult patients who have cancer will require an understanding of the role of aging, comorbidity, functional status, and frailty on treatment outcomes. The incorporation of CGA into the care of older patients who have cancer will ensure that the heterogeneity of this population is considered in the development of treatment plans. It also may improve outcomes by identifying and optimally treating comorbid conditions and functional impairments. Optimal treatment of the older adult patient who has cancer starts with careful delineation of goals through conversation. The treatment plan should be comprehensive and address cancer-specific treatment, symptom-specific treatment, supportive treatment modalities, and end-of-life care.

References

[1] Balducci L, Repetto L. Increased risk of myelotoxicity in elderly patients with Non-Hodgkin Lymphoma: The case for routine prophylaxis with colony-stimulating factor beginning in the first cycle of chemotherapy. Cancer 2004;100(1):6–11.

[2] Lindeman RD, Tobin J, Shock NW. Longitudinal studies on the rate of decline in renal function with age. J Am Geriatr Soc 1985;33:278–85.

[3] United States Corporate Athletic Association. Marathon Records by Age Group. Available at http://www.uscaa.org/marathon/records.htm. Accessed April 15, 2006.

[4] Jacobson SD, Cha S, Sargent DJ, et al. Tolerability, dose intensity and benefit of 5FU based chemotherapy for advanced colorectal cancer (CRC) in the elderly. Proc Am Soc Clin Oncol 2001;20:384a, abstract 1534.

[5] Wasil T, Lichtman SM. Clinical pharmacology issues relevant to the dosing and toxicity of chemotherapy in the elderly. Oncologist 2005;10:602–12.

[6] O'Mahoney MS, George G, Westlake H, et al. Plasma aspirin esterase activity in elderly patients undergoing elective hip replacement and with fractured neck of femur. Age Ageing 1994;23:338–41.

[7] Wynne HA, Cope LH, Herd B, et al. The association of age and frailty with paracetamol conjugation in man. Age Ageing 1990;19:419–24.

[8] Jacobs JR, Reves JG, Marty J, et al. Aging increases pharmacodynamic sensitivity to the hypnotic effects of midazolam. Anesth Analg 1995;80:143–8.

[9] Blasco MA. Telomeres and human disease: ageing, cancer and beyond. Nat Rev Genet 2005; 6:611–22.

[10] Cohen HJ. Oncology and aging: general principles of cancer in the elderly. In: Hazzard WR, Blass JP, Halter JB, et al, editors. Principles of geriatric medicine and gerontology. 5th edition. New York: McGraw-Hill; 2003. p. 673–5.

[11] Balducci L, Extermann M. Management of cancer in the older person: a practical approach. Oncologist 2000;5:224–37.

[12] Extermann M, Aapro M, Bernabei R, et al. Use of comprehensive geriatric assessment in older cancer patients: recommendations from the task force on CGA of the International Society of Geriatric Oncology. Crit Rev Oncol Hem 2005;55:241–52.

[13] Solomon D, Brown AS, Brummel-Smith K, et al. National Institutes of Health Consensus Development Conference statement: geriatric assessment methods for clinical decision-making. J Am Geriatr Soc 1988;36:342–7.

[14] Stuck AE, Siu AL, Wieland GD, et al. Comprehensive geriatric assessment: a meta-analysis of controlled trials. Lancet 1993;342:1032–6.
[15] Stuck AE, Egger M, Hammer A, et al. Home visits to prevent nursing home admission and functional declinein elderly people: systematic review and meta-regression analysis. JAMA 2002;287:1022–8.
[16] Reuben DB, Frank JC, Hirsch SH, et al. A randomized clinical trial of outpatient comprehensive geriatric assessment coupled with an intervention to increase adherence to recommendations. J Am Geriatr Soc 1999;47(3):269–76.
[17] Cohen HJ, Feussner JR, Weinberger M, et al. A controlled trial of inpatient and outpatient geriatric evaluation and management. N Engl J Med 2002;346:905–12.
[18] Rich MW, Beckham VT, Wittenburg C, et al. A multidisciplinary intervention to prevent the readmission of elderly patients with congestive heart failure. N Engl J Med 1995;333:1190–5.
[19] Rao AV, Hsieh F, Feussner JR, et al. Geriatric evaluation and management units in the care of the frail elderly cancer patient. J Gerontol: Med Sci 2005;60A:798–803.
[20] Ingram SS, Seo PH, Martell RE, et al. Comprehensive assessment of the elderly cancer patient: the feasibility of self-report methodology. J Clin Oncol 2002;20(3):770–5.
[21] Hurria A, Gupta S, Zauderer M, et al. Developing a cancer-specific geriatric assessment: a feasibility study. Cancer 2005;104:1998–2005.
[22] Extermann M, Meyer J, Mcginnis M, et al. A comprehensive geriatric intervention detects multiple problems in older breast cancer patients. Crit Rev Oncol Hematol 2004;49:69–75.
[23] Yancik R, Wesley MN, Ries LA, et al. Comorbidity and age as predictors of risk for early mortality of male and female colon carcinoma patients: a population-based study. Cancer 1998;82(11):2123–34.
[24] Yancik R, Wesley MN, Ries LA, et al. Effect of age and comorbidity in postmenopausal breast cancer patients aged 55 years and older. JAMA 2001;285(7):885–92.
[25] Passick SD, Dugan W, McDonald MV, et al. Oncologists' recognition of depression in their patients with cancer. J Clin Oncol 1998;16(4):1594–600.
[26] Chodosh J, Petitti DB, Elliot M, et al. Physician recognition of cognitive impairment: evaluating the need for improvement. J Am Geriatr Soc 2004;52(7):1051–9.
[27] Extermann M, Overcash J, Lyman GH, et al. Comorbidity and functional status are independent in older cancer patients. J Clin Oncol 1998;16(4):1582–7.
[28] Repetto L, Fratino L, Audisio RA, et al. Comprehensive geriatric assessment adds information to Eastern Cooperative Oncology Group performance status in elderly cancer patients: an Italian Group for Geriatric Oncology Study. J Clin Oncol 2002;20(2):494–502.
[29] Fried LP, Tangen CM, Walston J, et al. Cardiovascular Health Study Collaborative Research Group. Frailty in older adults: evidence for a phenotype. J Gerontol A Biol Sci Med Sci 2001;56(3):M146–56.
[30] Ferrucci L, Guralnik JM, Cavazzini C, et al. The frailty syndrome: a critical issue in geriatric oncology. Crit Rev Oncol Hematol 2003;46:127–37.
[31] Balducci L, Stanta G. Cancer in the frail patient: a coming epidemic. Hematol Oncol Clin North Am 2000;14:235–50.
[32] Audisio RA, Osman N, Audisio MM, et al. How do we manage breast cancer in the elderly patients? A survey among members of the British Association of Surgical Oncologists. Crit Rev Oncol Hematol 2004;52:135–41.
[33] Biganzoli L, Goldhirsch A, Straehle C, et al. Adjuvant chemotherapy in elderly patients with breast cancer: a survey of the British International Group. Annal Oncol 2004;15:207–10.
[34] Saliba D, Elliott M, Rubenstein LZ, et al. The Vulnerable Elders Survey: a tool for identifying vulnerable older people in the community. J Am Geriatr Soc 2001;49(12):1691–9.
[35] Monson K, Litvak DA, Bold RJ. Surgery in the aged population: surgical oncology. Arch Surg 2003;138(10):1061–7.
[36] Muss H, Woolf S, Berry D, et al. Cancer and leukemia group B. Adjuvant chemotherapy in older and younger women with lymph node-positive breast cancer. JAMA 2005;293(9):1073–81.

[37] Rose JH, O'Toole EE, Dawson NV, et al. Perspectives, preferences, care practices, and outcomes among older and middle-aged patients with late-stage cancer. J Clin Oncol 2004; 22(24):4907–17.
[38] Rao A, Cohen HJ. Symptom management in the elderly cancer patient: fatigue, pain, and depression. J Natl Cancer Inst Monogr 2004;32:150–7.
[39] Bukberg J, Penman D, Holland JC. Depression in hospitalized cancer patients. Psychosom Med 1984;46:199–212.
[40] Hopwood P, Stephens RJ. Depression in patients with lung cancer: prevalence and risk factors derived from quality-of-life data. J Clin Oncol 2000;18(4):893–903.
[41] Cassileth BR, Lusk EJ, Brown LL, et al. Factors associated with psychological distress in cancer patients. Med Pediatr Oncol 1986;14:251–4.
[42] Roberts RE, Vernon SW. The Center for Epidemiologica Studies Depression Scale: its use in a community sample. Am J Psychiatry 1983;140:41–6.
[43] Montorio I, Izal M. The Geriatric Depression Scale: a review of its development and utility. Int Psychogeriatr 1996;8:103–12.
[44] Koenig HG, Cohen HJ, Blazer DG, et al. A brief depression scale for use in the medically ill. Int J Psychiatry Med 1992;22:183–95.
[45] Demark-Wahnefried W, Morey MC, Clipp EC, et al. Leading the way in exercise and diet (Project LEAD): intervening to improve function among older breast and prostate cancer survivors. Control Clin Trials 2003;24:206–23.
[46] Demark-Wahnefried W, Aziz NM, Rowland JH, et al. Riding the crest of the teachable moment: promoting long-term health after the diagnosis of cancer. J Clin Oncol 2005;23(24): 5814–30.
[47] Ingram SS, Seo PH, Sloane R, et al. The association between oral health and general health and quality if life in older male cancer patients. J Am Geriatr Soc 2005;53:1504–9.
[48] Hewitt M, Rowland JH, Yancik R. Cancer survivors in the United States: age, health, and disability. J Gerontol A Biol Sci Med Sci 2003;58(1):82–91.
[49] Clipp EC, Hollis DR, Cohen HJ. Considerations of psychosocial illness phase in cancer survival. Psychooncology 2001;10(2):166–78.
[50] Haley WE. The costs of family caregiving: implications for geriatric oncology. Crit Rev Oncol Hematol 2003;48(2):151–8.
[51] Sutton LM, Demark-Wahnefried W, Clipp EC. Management of terminal cancer in elderly patients. Lancet Oncol 2003;4(3):149–57.
[52] Lewis JH, Kilgore ML, Goldman DP, et al. Participation of patients 65 years of age or older in cancer clinical trials. J Clin Oncol 2003;21:1383–9.
[53] Kemeny MM, Peterson BL, Kornblith AB, et al. Wheeler J. Levine E. Bartlett N. Fleming G. Cohen HJ. Barriers to clinical trial participation by older women with breast cancer. J Clin Oncol 2003;21(12):2268–75.
[54] Kornblith AB, Kemeny M, Peterson BL, et al. Cancer and leukemia group B. Survey of oncologists' perceptions of barriers to accrual of older patients with breast carcinoma to clinical trials. Cancer 2002;95(5):989–96.
[55] Yancik R. Integration of aging and cancer research in geriatric medicine. J Gerontol A Biol Sci Med Sci 1997;52(6):M329–32.
[56] Balducci L. Geriatric oncology. Crit Rev Oncol Hematol 2003;46:211–20.
[57] Monfardini S. Geriatric oncology: a new subspecialty? J Clin Oncol 2004;22(22):4655.
[58] Mathias S, Nayak US, Isaacs B. Balance in elderly patients: the "get-up and go" test. Arch Phys Med Rehabil 1986;67(6):387–9.

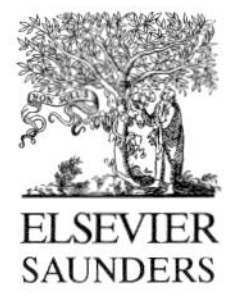

ELSEVIER
SAUNDERS

NURSING CLINICS OF NORTH AMERICA

Nurs Clin N Am 43 (2008) 323–327

Index

Note: Page numbers of article titles are in **boldface** type.

doi:10.1016/S0029-6465(08)00030-3

I

L

M

N

O

P

R

S

T

W

Oncology nursing:
past, present, and future: